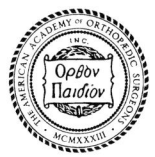
American Academy of Orthopaedic Surgeons
6300 North River Road
Rosemont, Illinois 60018
1-800-626-6726

Total Shoulder Arthroplasty

EDITED BY
LYNN A. CROSBY, MD, FACS
Professor
Director of Shoulder Surgery
Department of Orthopaedic Surgery
Wright State University School of Medicine
Dayton, Ohio

CONTRIBUTORS
Julian S. Arroyo, MD
Louis Bigliani, MD
R. Michael Gross, MD
James M. Hill, MD
Geoffrey Johnston, MD
William M. Levine, MD
J. Michael Wiater, MD

SERIES EDITOR
Thomas R. Johnson, MD

Board of Directors 2000

S. Terry Canale, MD
President

Richard H. Gelberman, MD
Vernon T. Tolo, MD
William J. Robb, III, MD
Andrew J. Weiland, MD
Robert D. D'Ambrosia, MD
James D. Heckman, MD
Joseph P. Iannotti, MD, PHD
Ramon L. Jimenez, MD
Darren L. Johnson, MD
Thomas P. Sculco, MD
John R. Tongue, MD
David A. Halsey, MD
Lowry Jones, Jr., MD
Richard B. Welch, MD
Gary E. Friedlaender, MD
William W. Tipton, Jr., MD (Ex Officio)

Vice-President, Educational Programs
Mark W. Wieting

Director, Department of Publications
Marilyn L. Fox, PhD

Managing Editor
Lynne Roby Shindoll

Manager, Manufacturing and Sales
Paul D. Psilos, PhD

Assistant Production Manager
Sophie Tosta

Editorial Assistant
Anu Amaran

Production Assistants
Karen Danca
Shawn Singer

The American Academy of Orthopaedic Surgeons Monograph Series is dedicated to Wendy O. Schmidt, American Academy of Orthopaedic Surgeons senior medical editor, 1987-1991.

TOTAL SHOULDER ARTHROPLASTY
American Academy of Orthopaedic Surgeons

The material presented in *Total Shoulder Arthroplasty* has been made available by the American Academy of Orthopaedic Surgeons for educational purposes only. This material is not intended to present the only, or necessarily best, methods or procedures for the medical situations discussed, but rather is intended to represent an approach, view, statement, or opinion of the author(s) or producer(s), which may be helpful to others who face similar situations.

Some drugs or medical devices demonstrated in Academy print or electronic publications have not been cleared by the Food and Drug Administration (FDA) or have been cleared by the FDA for specific uses only. The FDA has stated that it is the responsibility of the physician to determine the FDA clearance status of each drug or device he or she wishes to use in clinical practice.

Furthermore, any statements about commercial products are solely the opinion of the author(s) and do not represent an Academy endorsement or evaluation of these products. These statements may not be used in advertising or for any commercial purpose.

All rights reserved. No part of this publication may be reproduced, stored in a retrieval system, or transmitted, in any form, or by any means, electronic, mechanical, photocopying, recording, or otherwise, without prior written permission from the publisher.

First Edition
Copyright © 2000 by the
American Academy of Orthopaedic Surgeons

ISBN 0-89203-235-9

CONTENTS

PREFACE	vii
THE HISTORY OF TOTAL SHOULDER ARTHROPLASTY	1
INDICATIONS	17
SURGICAL TECHNIQUE AND RESULTS	27
COMPLICATIONS	39
REVISION SHOULDER ARTHROPLASTY	47
FUTURE DIRECTIONS	65
INDEX	69

CONTRIBUTORS

Julian S. Arroyo, MD
Lakewood Orthopaedic Surgeons
Lakewood, Washington

Louis Bigliani, MD
Professor and Chairman
Department of Orthopaedic Surgery
Columbia University
New York, New York

Lynn A. Crosby, MD, FACS
Professor
Director of Shoulder Surgery
Department of Orthopaedic Surgery
Wright State University School of Medicine
Dayton, Ohio

R. Michael Gross, MD
Assistant Clinical Professor Orthopaedic Surgery
Creighton University/University of Nebraska Medical Center
Omaha, Nebraska

James M. Hill, MD
Orthopaedic Associates
Arlington Heights, Illinois

Geoffrey Johnston, MD
Professor of Orthopaedic Surgery
University of Saskatchewan
Saskatoon, Saskatchewan, Canada

William H. Levine, MD
Assistant Attending
The Shoulder Service
Director, Sports Medicine
Orthopaedic Surgery
Columbia-Presbyterian Medical Center
New York, New York

J. Michael Wiater, MD
Shoulder Fellow
The Shoulder Service
New York Orthopaedic Hospital
Columbia-Presbyterian Medical Campus
New York Presbyterian Hospital
New York, New York

PREFACE

I would like to dedicate this monograph to Dr. Douglas Harryman, who passed away December 24, 1999, after a long and courageous fight with osteosarcoma. He was an educator, researcher, surgeon, husband, father, athlete, and most of all, a friend who will be missed dearly by all who knew him.

Replacement surgery of the shoulder joint is becoming more common but probably will never be performed as often as knee or hip arthroplasty. Shoulder surgery has become more specialized over the past 10 years, with more orthopaedic surgeons dedicating their practices to the care of the shoulder joint. Replacement surgery of the shoulder is now being taught in most orthopaedic residency programs, and with a growing number of postgraduate fellowships available, the care of shoulder-related problems is improving rapidly. This monograph is an attempt to present the most current information on this challenging procedure.

The monograph, however, does not address every nuance of the current art of shoulder replacement. Space simply does not allow us to consider attempting such a lofty goal. Rather, I asked R. Michael Gross to review the history of shoulder arthroplasty to give the reader an appreciation of where this procedure started and how it has progressed over time. James Hill discusses the current indications for shoulder replacement. The technique of primary replacement therapy was written by Julian Arroyo, and the expert tutelage of his mentors, Louis Bigliani and Evan Flatow, is clearly apparent in his contribution. My contribution was to detail the complications that, unfortunately, are far too common with this procedure. Surgeons must anticipate potential complications in order to avoid them and advise patients about the possibility of complications so that they will not be disappointed and discouraged when a complication does occur. The challenges associated with revision shoulder arthroplasty are described by J. Michael Wiater and William Levine. Their chapter is an exceptional work that provides helpful advice about treating a failed shoulder replacement to obtain results that will benefit the patient with adequate pain relief. The monograph concludes with Geoffrey Johnston and Louis Bigliani writing candidly about the future of shoulder arthroplasty and the major improvements we as surgeons can expect.

I want to acknowledge Sophie Tosta, Assistant Production Manager, who has made my job as editor a truly enjoyable experience. Also a special thank you to Lynne Shindoll, Managing Editor, whom I have had the pleasure of working with on previous Academy projects and whose experience and expert judgment are, in my opinion, irreplaceable.

Finally, I want to thank my wife Sheila, daughters Shanna and Allison, and son Ryan for allowing me the time to take on this project. Without their continued support and understanding of the extra time spent at my desk, this monograph would not have been possible.

LYNN A. CROSBY, MD

THE HISTORY OF TOTAL SHOULDER ARTHROPLASTY

R. MICHAEL GROSS, MD

The first shoulder replacement arthroplasty was performed in 1893 by Jules Emil Péan[1-3] (Fig. 1). His procedure followed closely on the heels of a report in 1890 by Themistockles Gluck of using custom ivory hemiarthroplasties to reconstruct the knee, elbow, and wrist joints.[4] Gluck also was reported to have designed, but not implanted, an ivory shoulder joint.[5] Péan's operation differed from Gluck's in that it was a total joint replacement. His patient, a 37-year-old baker, had extensive tuberculosis of the proximal humerus. Although the patient refused the only available treatment at the time, an amputation, he agreed to an experimental operation consisting of excision of the infected bone and replacement with an artificial joint. The appliance, constructed of platinum and a hardened rubber ball trapped between rings attached to the humeral and glenoid components (Fig. 2), was designed and fabricated by Péan's dentist, J. Porter Michaels.

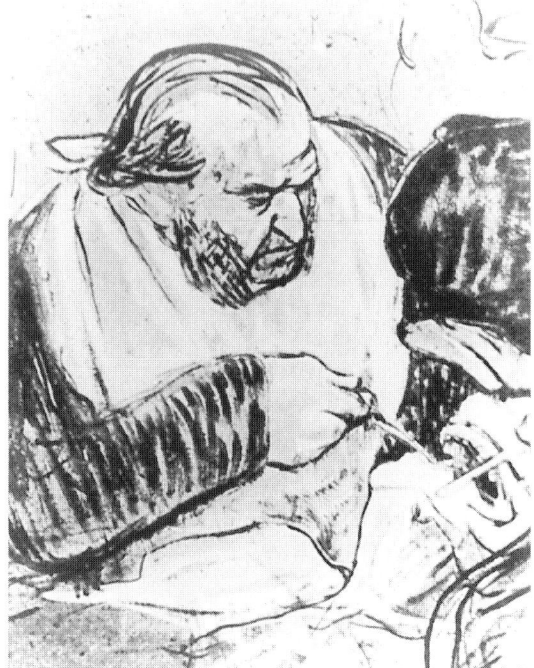

FIGURE 1
A portrait of Jules Emile Péan (1830–1898) painted by Henri Toulouse-Lautrec. (Reproduced with permission from Lugli T: Artificial shoulder joint by Péan (1893). Clin Orthop 1978; 133:215–218.)

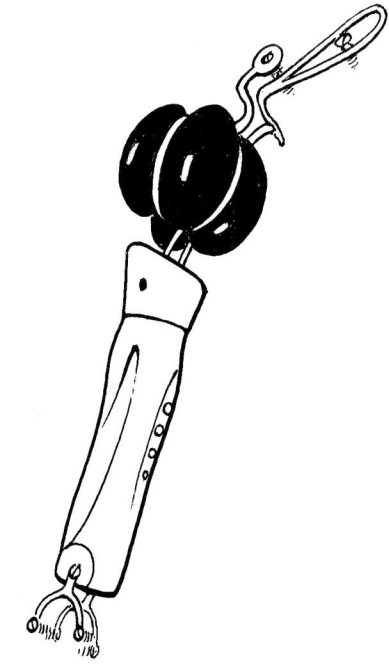

FIGURE 2
Prosthesis implanted by Péan in 1893. This appliance, which is on exhibit at the Smithsonian Institution, was the first shoulder joint ever implanted and probably the first total joint arthroplasty of any type.

Remarkably, this two-step procedure was successful for several years[6] before the infection recurred and the appliance had to be removed.

As remarkable and modern as Péan's operation was, it was actually an aberration in the development of joint arthroplasty that began with the work of John Rhea Barton in 1826. Barton's initial work was aimed at mobilizing a malpositioned stiff hip—a relatively common problem in his time. His classic article[7] describes a 21-year-old Irish sailor, who fell 6 or 7 feet from the hatchway into the ship's hold, injuring his right hip. Following the injury, the sailor was unable to walk and the hip became rigidly fixed in a flexed position. The patient was seen by Barton 7 months after the injury and he hospitalized him for an additional year, trying all available means, yet failing to mobilize the joint. Barton then proposed an osteotomy of the hip to allow range of motion and promote a "functional pseudoarthrosis." This procedure, carried out on November 22, 1826, as a 7-minute operation, was the first true joint arthroplasty.

In 1867, Louis Xavier Edouard Leopold Ollier[8] built on Barton's success, by performing in vitro studies of the interposition of soft tissue at an osteotomy site to ensure a functional pseudoarthrosis. The significance of Barton's and Ollier's work was recognized by John B. Murphy[9] who applied it clinically. Murphy reported on his experience with 84 arthroplasties of various joints, including the shoulder joint, using Ollier's technique with the insertion of local flaps of fascia and fatty tissue.[10]

Murphy's success was expanded on by William Baer,[11] who presented to the American Orthopedic Association his extensive experience using free fascial flaps composed of chromicized pig bladder, a foreign but adsorbable material similar to chromic suture. This approach equaled the success of local flaps; however, it had an advantage in that it could be done through a smaller incision and was less difficult for the surgeon. In their 1929 book,[12] Russell and Andrew MacAusland detailed Baer's and other current methods of arthroplasty. In addition, they defined the parameters for a successful arthroplasty, giving equal weight to motion, pain relief, and stability: "The true test for an Arthroplasty lies in positive answers to the following questions: is there sufficient motion in the joint to increase function? Is the motion painless? Is the joint stable? Any arthroplasty that does not measure up to these requirements is not a success."[12]

MacAusland described a technique for shoulder arthroplasty through the use of free flaps to provide painless, stable shoulder motion. This procedure rarely was used, because at that time the primary indication for an arthroplasty was ankylosis of a joint or combination of joints causing a severe functional disability. The shoulder, with its scapulothoracic motion, was much more forgiving, making the need for arthroplasty rare. However, the MacAusland interposition shoulder arthroplasty has endured, and it currently is used occasionally as an alternative type of arthroplasty under unusual circumstances.[13] Interposition arthroplasty persisted as the standard into the early 1930s, when it was replaced by more effective procedures. It is fascinating to note that the problems Murphy faced almost 100 years ago remain today. He was concerned with the importance of strict asepsis during surgery. He notes: "If (a) sepsis does occur, the entire procedure is likely to be nullified."[9]

Marius Nygaard Smith-Petersen contributed the next advance in the development of joint arthroplasty by returning to Gluck's approach of using a foreign, nonadsorbable material. This step, as related by Peltier,[6] was taken when in 1923 Smith-Petersen noticed that a foreign body reaction to a piece of glass caused a smooth synovial sac. He applied this principle to the concept of degenerative arthritis of the hip and moved from glass to Vitallium in the development of the cup, or mold, arthroplasty. This procedure remained the treatment of choice for hip arthritis for the next 30 years, and it led to the development of a shoulder cup arthroplasty,[14] first by E. Jónsson (Fig. 3) and later by Varian,[15] who used a Silastic cup. The latter procedure was short-lived as a result of its marginal success and high complication rate.

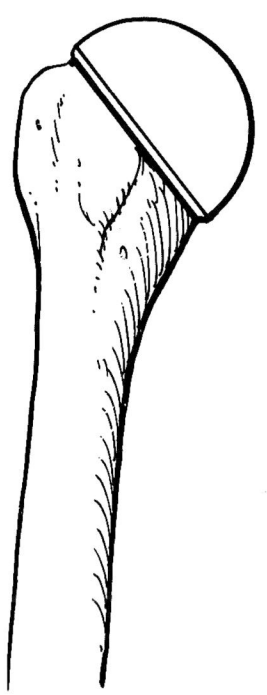

FIGURE 3
Cup arthroplasty. The Jónsson shoulder cup was an extrapolation of the Smith Peterson cup arthroplasty for the hip to the problem of shoulder arthritis. The initial cups were simply Smith Peterson hip cups; only later were they specifically designed for the shoulder.

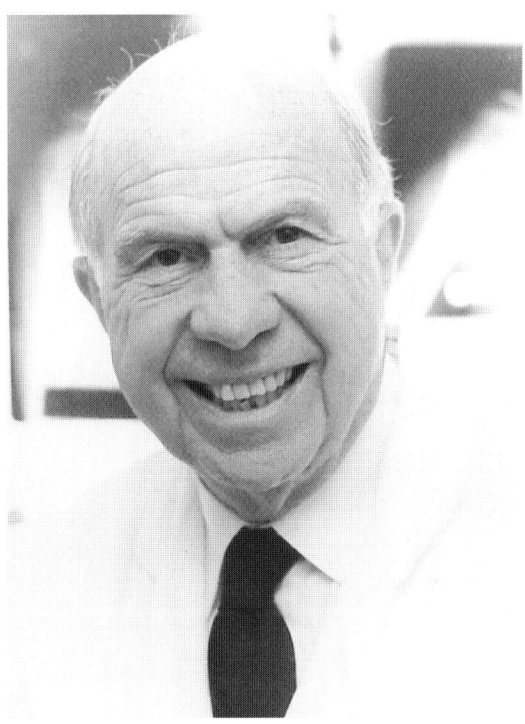

FIGURE 4
Charles S. Neer, II. (Photo by Bill Mitchell Photography, Paramus, NJ. Courtesy of Charles S. Neer, II.)

From the late 1930s through the early 1950s, a number of appliances were developed for the treatment not only of degenerative joint disease but also of fractures. Most of this research was aimed at the hip. However, in 1951 Krueger[16] reported on the use of an anatomically designed humeral head prosthesis for the treatment of osteonecrosis. In 1952, Richard and associates[17] reported on Judet's use of an acrylic appliance to replace the proximal humerus in a case of fracture-dislocation of the shoulder. In 1953, deAnquin, from Argentina, also inserted an acrylic humeral appliance.[18] It is not clear why Krueger's approach did not become more popular, whereas the acrylic appliances appeared to have been rejected as a result of design flaws as well as problems with the durability of the material.[19]

In 1953, Charles S. Neer, II (Fig. 4) and associates[20] reported on the treatment of comminuted fracture-dislocations of the proximal humerus. This article introduced the possibility of using a humeral endoprosthesis to improve the results of the treatment for this difficult fracture. In 1955, Neer[21] reported his experience in treating this fracture as well as posttraumatic arthritis with an endoprosthesis, known as the Neer I (Fig. 5). Neer's short-term results, in which 11 of the 12 patients were pain-free, provided momentum to extend the study and expand the indications for shoulder replacement. In 1964, he published a 2- to 11-year follow-up for an expanded group of 42 patients, including some with degenerative joint disease.[22] His work was the index research that moved humeral replacement into mainstream orthopaedics.

John Charnley was the next major influence on shoulder arthroplasty through his work on the treatment of hip arthritis. The three areas that he

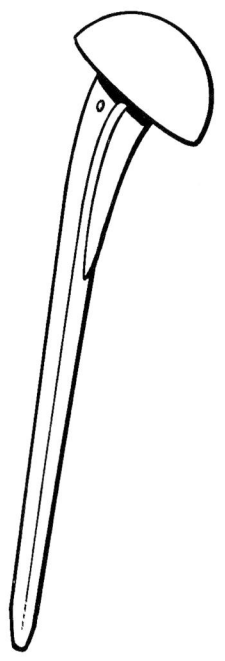

FIGURE 5
The Neer I humeral prosthesis. The use of this appliance situated humeral replacement into mainstream orthopaedics.

championed were: (1) taking steps to lower the infection rate; (2) fixation of the appliance with acrylic cement; and (3) low-friction total joint replacement through the use of a high-density polyethylene liner.

Charnley's work had an enormous impact on all major joint reconstructions. By the early 1970s, several authors[23–26] reported on the use of polyethylene with a humeral prosthesis; thus, for the first time since 1893, attention returned to Péan's initial approach of a total shoulder joint replacement. Charnley's success led to an explosive growth in the development of many prosthetic replacement joints, including the shoulder. As often as not, the research was driven by the surgeon's intuition rather than biomechanics.

The early shoulder appliances met two of the MacAuslands'[12] three principles for a successful arthroplasty. These appliances could deal with the issues of freedom from pain and adequate motion; however, the element of stability proved to be a continual problem. This problem was dealt with by adding constraint into the shoulder systems. With the addition of these new designs, total shoulder systems were classified as one of three general types (Table 1): unconstrained, semiconstrained, and constrained.

The unconstrained systems relied on the normal anatomy of the shoulder joint to provide stability while the prosthesis itself was directed more to the problems of mobility and pain relief. These systems frequently overlapped with the semiconstrained systems, because increased constraint could be an option within the same system, depending on what type of glenoid component was inserted. Neer (in conjunction with Robert G. Averill) led the way with the first complete unconstrained total shoulder system, the Neer II, introduced in 1973 (Fig. 6). During the next 8 years, the Neer II system was field tested as directed by the United States Food and Drug Administration before it was released for general use. During that time a variety of glenoid components were also tested, including different thicknesses, different anchoring systems, augmentations to account for glenoid wear, and semiconstrained hooded components (referred to as the 200% and 600% glenoids) for added stability. Neer[18] states that in his most recent series of 408 shoulders followed for more than 2 years, only three shoulders had to undergo reoperation for glenoid loosening. He further states that the standard polyethylene glenoid component remains preferred. The Neer II system remains in popular use today.

The Neer II was followed in Europe in 1975 by a system designed by Engelbrecht and Stellbrink[23] called the St. Georg (Fig. 7). The St. Georg was initially developed as a polyethylene liner to articulate with the Neer appliance, but later a spherical humeral component with various unconstrained and semiconstrained glenoid components was developed. The high rate of glenoid loosening experienced by Engelbrecht and Stellbrink led them to return in 1979 to prosthetic replacement of the humeral head alone without resurfacing the glenoid. With the discontinuation of the glenoid component, Engelbrecht and

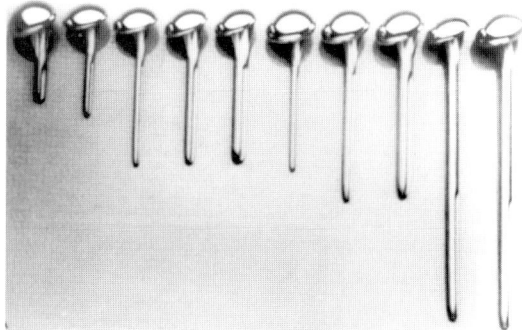

FIGURE 6
The Neer II system. The articular surface of the head was rounded to avoid damage to the polyethylene glenoid. The radius of curvature remained 44 mm and matched that of the glenoid. A second head length was added as well as a variety of stems to offer greater versatility. (Courtesy of Charles S. Neer, II.)

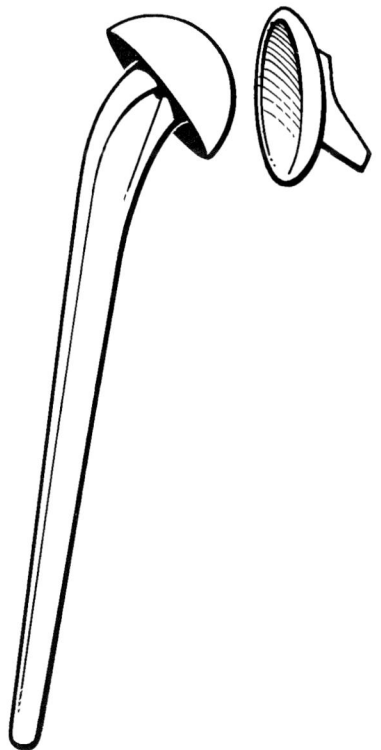

FIGURE 7
The St. Georg. Initially this was no more than a polyethylene glenoid matched to a Neer I appliance. Later, an entire system was developed with a variety of constraints built into the glenoid component.

Stellbrink began to perform adjunctive procedures on the glenoid to improve the results of hemiarthroplasty. The aim of glenoidplasties, was to increase the surface area of the articulation as well as to improve the stability of the glenohumeral joint by buttressing the humeral head prosthesis against loads directed superomedially without adding a glenoid component. These changes could consist of glenoid osteotomy and cancellous bone graft, glenoid roof augmentation, or glenoid deepening.[27]

The DANA (designed after natural anatomy), also known as the University of California at Los Angeles (UCLA) total shoulder (Fig. 8), was designed by Ian Clarke in collaboration with Harlan C. Amstutz. This design, introduced in 1976, was similar to the St. Georg insofar as it was both unconstrained and semiconstrained. In 1988, Amstutz and associates[28] reported on a group of 56 DANA arthroplasties with a minimum of 2 years of follow-up. Eleven percent of the unconstrained appliances required revision, whereas 20% of the hooded glenoids required revision. The authors advised against abduction past 90° in any rotator cuff-deficient shoulder that has been repaired with a hooded glenoid. The results were somewhat disappointing, yet the authors were optimistic that the DANA was a better overall solution when compared with any constrained appliance.

In 1981, the Monospherical (Fig. 9), also known as the Gristina, was introduced. This appliance had slightly more constraint built in the glenoid than did the Neer, and it required greater resection of the humeral head compared with any of the previous unconstrained appliances. The slightly over-hemispherical head increased the mechanical advantage of the deltoid and rotator cuff and allowed for increased motion, whereas the glenoid offered a slight amount of dorsal support to increase stability. In 1987, Gristina and associates[29] reported on 100 total shoulder arthroplasties followed for an average of 38.2 months (range, 6 to 73 months). Ninety percent attained good or excellent pain relief. These authors reported increases in shoulder motion, particularly in active abduction and

TABLE 1
FAMILY TREE

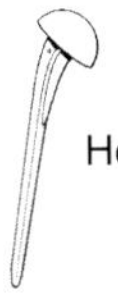

```
    Neer* 1951                        Péan* 1893
Hemiarthroplasty-Unconstrained    Total Shoulder Arthroplasty
                                       (TSA)-Constrained
        └──── Humeral endoprosthesis ─────┴──── Charnley-THA ────
```

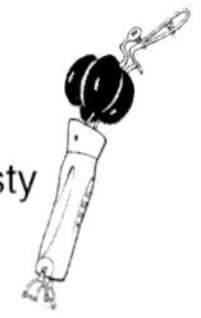

Unconstrained

Neer II (Neer clones)
Designed to reproduce normal anatomy... Endo or TSA.

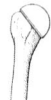
Cup Arthroplasty
<u>Jónsson</u> (metal), <u>Varian</u>, (Silastic Cup), <u>O'Leary-Walker</u> (metal) included an optional glenoid component.

DANA (UCLA) & Monospherical (Gristina)
Systems require greater bone resection and have more constraint built into the glenoid component.

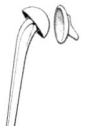
St. Georg
Primarily used in Europe...Endo or TSA.

Isoelastic
Shoulder implant primarily European use... Endo or TSA.

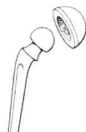
Bipolar
Bateman, Swanson, MacNab.
Forgiving appliance, fills the glenoid vault, theoretically offers more motion with less stress on the glenoid.

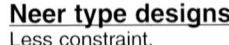

Neer type designs
Less constraint, modularity to offer better soft tissue balance and avoid eccentric loading of the glenoid...Press-fit, cemented, or bony ingrowth.

Bipolar
Designed to deal with extensive rotator cuff deficiencies or failed constrained TSAs.

In the end it appears that Neer's original design is as similar to the "modern TSA" as Charnley's initial THA is the the "modern THA."

Semiconstrained

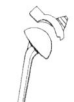
DANA (Designed After Natural Anatomy).
Hooded glenoid.

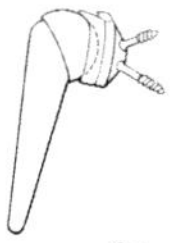

English-MacNab
Uncemented design.
Hooded with a deep glenoid.

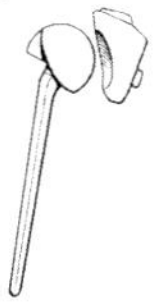

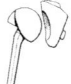
Mazas
This appliance exemplifies qualities of all three methods to semiconstrain a humeral endoprosthesis:
- Hooded.
- Glenoid physically attached to the acromion...acts like a spacer.
- The deep glenoid acts like a "bowl" to contain the humeral head.

Clayton "Spacer"
Polyethylene appliance designed to maintain the interval between the head and the acromion.

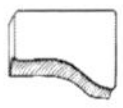

Neer hooded
Appliance...200% and 600% glenoid components.

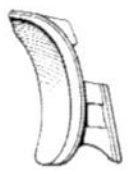

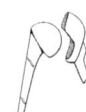
St. Georg hooded

Some of these appliances may still be available, however, they would be hard to find. There was a poor benefit risk ratio when one compares the functional improvement weighed against the increased complications.

*On display at the Smithsonian.

TOTAL SHOULDER ARTHROPLASTY

Since 1951 it is estimated that 70 "shoulder systems" have been developed. Most of these have been very short-lived. This tree is intended only to represent some of the more commonly used appliances, or those with unique characteristics. It is not meant to be all-inclusive nor to insult the "descendants" not represented in the tree.
-RMG

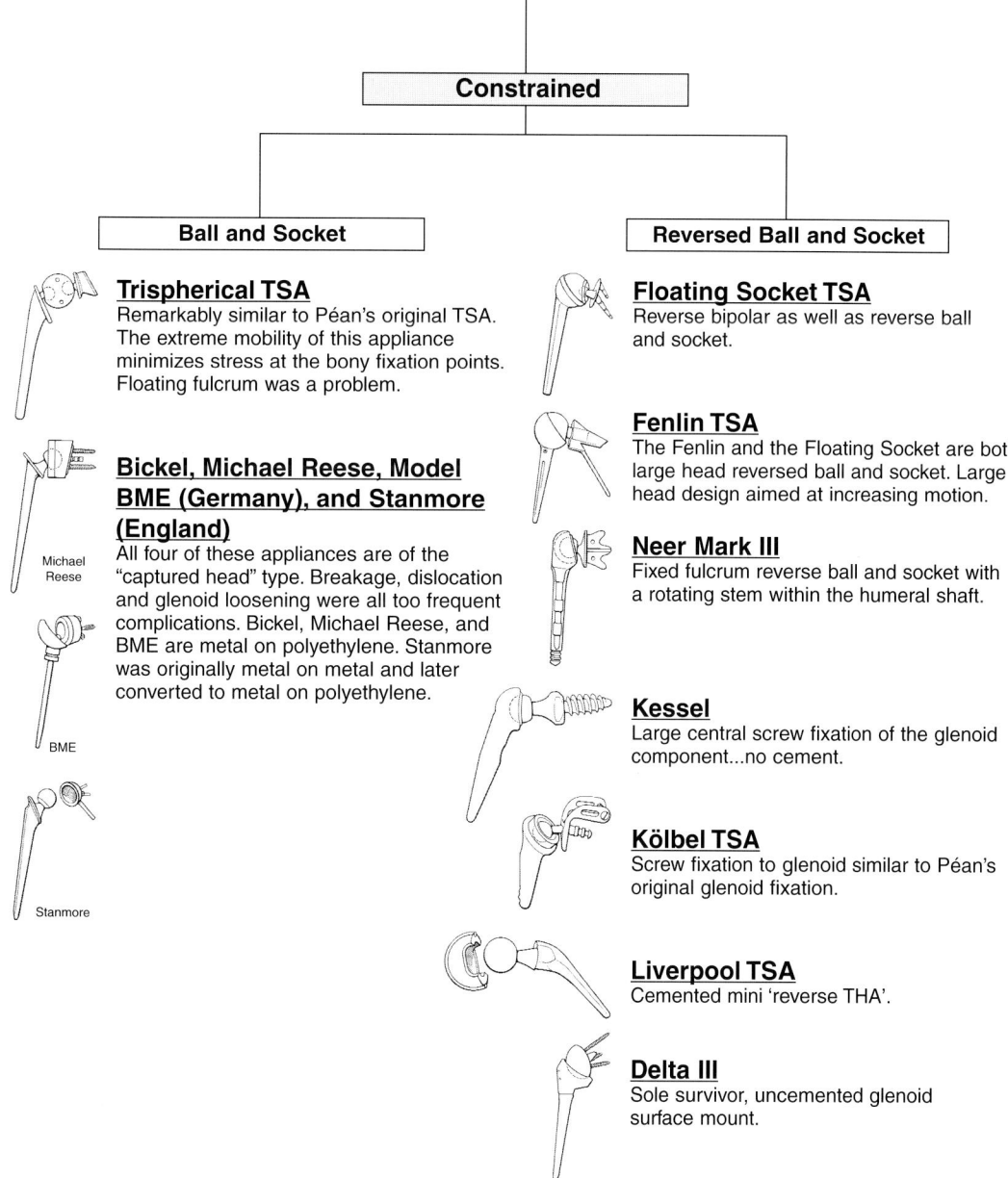

Constrained

Ball and Socket

Trispherical TSA
Remarkably similar to Péan's original TSA. The extreme mobility of this appliance minimizes stress at the bony fixation points. Floating fulcrum was a problem.

Bickel, Michael Reese, Model BME (Germany), and Stanmore (England)
All four of these appliances are of the "captured head" type. Breakage, dislocation and glenoid loosening were all too frequent complications. Bickel, Michael Reese, and BME are metal on polyethylene. Stanmore was originally metal on metal and later converted to metal on polyethylene.

Reversed Ball and Socket

Floating Socket TSA
Reverse bipolar as well as reverse ball and socket.

Fenlin TSA
The Fenlin and the Floating Socket are both large head reversed ball and socket. Large head design aimed at increasing motion.

Neer Mark III
Fixed fulcrum reverse ball and socket with a rotating stem within the humeral shaft.

Kessel
Large central screw fixation of the glenoid component...no cement.

Kölbel TSA
Screw fixation to glenoid similar to Péan's original glenoid fixation.

Liverpool TSA
Cemented mini 'reverse THA'.

Delta III
Sole survivor, uncemented glenoid surface mount.

Development as well as failure of the constrained TSA came as a result of two false assumptions–
   1) Most arthritic problems would have deficient rotator cuffs.
   2) The function of the rotator cuff could be effectively replaced by a fixed fulcrum.

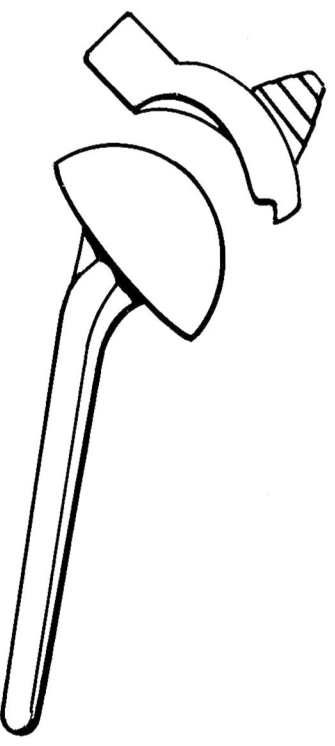

FIGURE 8
The designed after natural anatomy (DANA) also known as the University of California at Los Angeles (UCLA) shown with regular and hooded components.

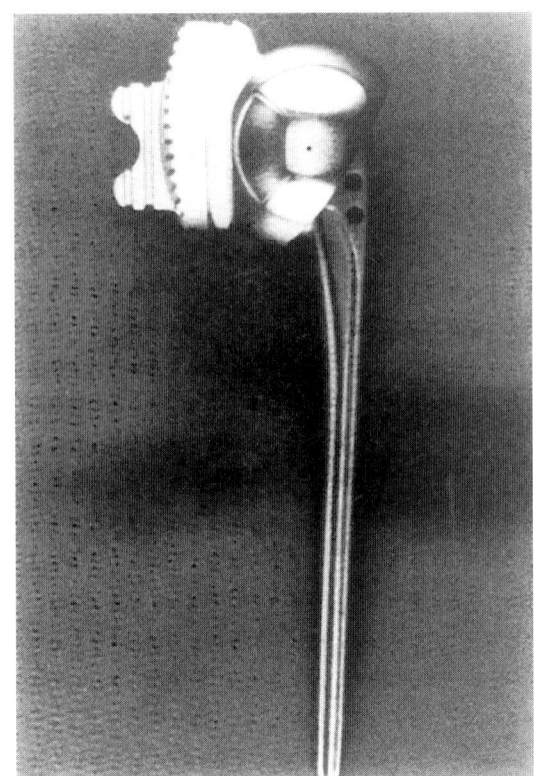

FIGURE 9
The Monospherical also known as the Gristina: This appliance had a slightly larger head to offer greater mobility and moderate constraint built into the glenoid component. (Reproduced with permission from Brenner B, Ferlic D, Clayton M, Dennis D: Survivorship of unconstrained total shoulder arthroplasty. J Bone Joint Surg 1989;71A:1289–1296.)

external rotation, in all patients, but the degree varied greatly within the diagnostic categories. They went on to state that the degree of postoperative shoulder motion achieved depended directly on the intraoperative condition of the rotator cuff and supporting soft tissue of the shoulder and that resection of the coracoacromial ligament is not indicated because it guides the rotator cuff and helps prevent superior subluxation. Both of these statements may be relatively obvious today, but they were significantly forward-thinking at the time they were made.

The semiconstrained devices offered increased stability to the shoulder joint by alternating the glenoid component in one of three ways. Some, such as the DANA, added a hood to the glenoid component. Others, such as the St. Georg, provided a bowl for the humerus by deepening the glenoid compartment. The Clayton spacer was a separate polyethylene component that could be attached to the acromion to prevent cephalad migration of the humeral head. The Mazas, from France, had characteristics of all three types of constraints. The glenoid was both deep and hooded as well as physically attached to the acromion. Mazas and de la Caffinière,[30] in reporting on 38 cases, found a relatively high complication rate and limited function. The quantity of bone in the glenoid vault is quite limited, and as a result, it is difficult to get durable fixation when any constraint is added to the glenoid component. The ideal case for the constrained or semi-

TABLE 2

HISTORY OF DEVELOPMENT OF CONSTRAINED DEVICES

Name of Device	Developer(s)	Year Developed/Introduced
Stanmore (Fig. 10)	Scales, Lettin	1969
Kölbel	Kölbel	1972
Bickel (Fig. 11)	Bickel	1972
BME	Zippel	1972
Neer Mark III (Fig. 12)	Neer, Averill	1972
Michael Reese	Post	1973
Kessel	Kessel	1973
Liverpool	Beddow, Elloy	1975
Fenlin	Fenlin	1975
Floating Socket (Fig. 13)	Buechel, Pappas, DePalma	1976
Tri-spherical (Fig. 14)	Gristina	1978
Delta III (Fig. 15)	Grammont	1990

constrained appliance was a rotator cuff-deficient shoulder; if the rotator cuff was present, it was very difficult to get adequate closure to allow for normal rotator cuff function with the large glenoid component in place. As later found by Franklin and associates,[31] rotator cuff insufficiency frequently leads to eccentric loading of the glenoid, creating a "rocking horse" effect that produces loosening of the glenoid component in a high percentage of cases. The combination of poor performance with a high complication rate has reduced the interest in these semiconstrained devices.

The constrained devices were the most aggressive designs. They were based on the presumption that the function of the rotator cuff could be replaced by a mechanical fixed fulcrum. A wide variety of these devices were introduced. The approximate date that each was developed or introduced is given in Table 2.

The Stanmore was the first and certainly one of the more popular European constrained total shoulder arthroplasties[32] (Fig. 10). Its initial design mimicked a total hip arthroplasty; however, it was metal on metal. The humeral ball initially was not captured and could dislocate. Later, when a polyethylene liner was added, the head was locked into the glenoid and it became more constrained. As with other constrained total shoulder arthroplasties, indications for its use were limited. Functional results failed to meet expectations, and complications exceeded them. The Stanmore has seen very little use since 1980.

The Kölbel, created in 1972, was a reverse ball and socket design that demonstrated the clinical application of biomechanical principles. The

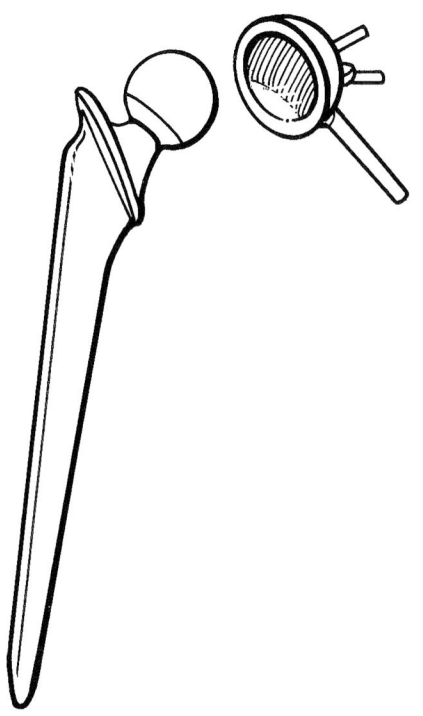

FIGURE 10
The Stanmore. One of the earliest total shoulder replacements. Initially it was highly semiconstrained with a metal on metal configuration. Later more constraint was added by capturing the ball with a polyethylene liner, which was added to the glenoid component.

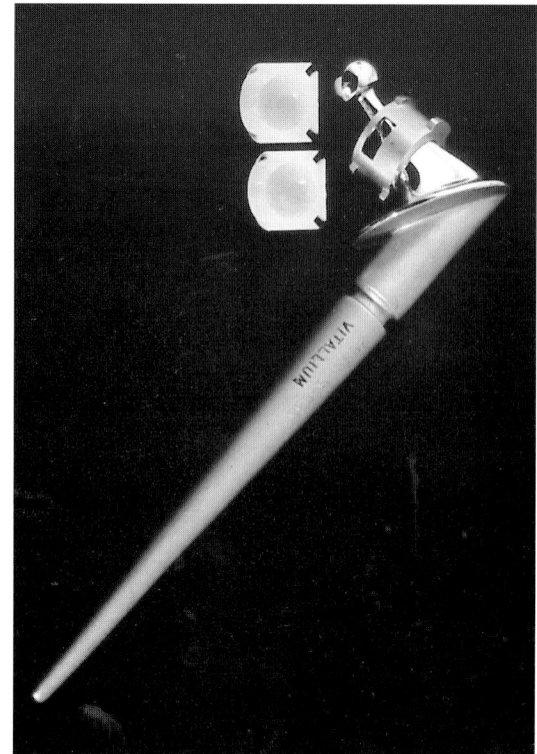

FIGURE 11
The Bickel. Appliance failure and loosening from its fixation in the glenoid vault led to its early demise. The large head of the screw uses the strong cortical bone for support. (Courtesy of Robert Cofield, Rochester, MN.)

scapular attachment, recognized as a weak link, was protected by attaching the appliance primarily to the cortical surface of the glenoid and also to the glenoid neck. As further protection, instability was designed into the appliance to protect the scapular attachment; when baseline torque was exceeded, the appliance would dislocate rather than cause failure of the anatomic anchor.

The Bickel (Fig. 11), the BME, and the Michael Reese were similar insofar as they were all captured ball and socket appliances. All three were underdesigned initially, resulting in material failure. The Bickel had a relatively short lifespan. In its trial of 12 cases from 1972 through 1975, complications of material failures and glenoid loosening, as well as limited function, led to its discontinuation.[33] Preliminary results of the BME reported in 1977 of 11 patients were classified as good; however, four prosthetic fractures occurred in the neck of the appliance on arthroplasties performed elsewhere.[34] This model never became popular and was discarded because of clinical problems.

The Michael Reese prothesis was designed by Melvin Post with modern biomechanical principles used in its development.[35–37] As with the Kölbel, Post's design recognized that the strength of the glenoid attachment was in its cortical surface and not in the glenoid vault. The glenoid component was surface mounted onto the cortical bone of the glenoid through a combination of a central peg and screws embedded in methylmethacrylate. Post also recognized that instability could protect the glenoid attachment and was an

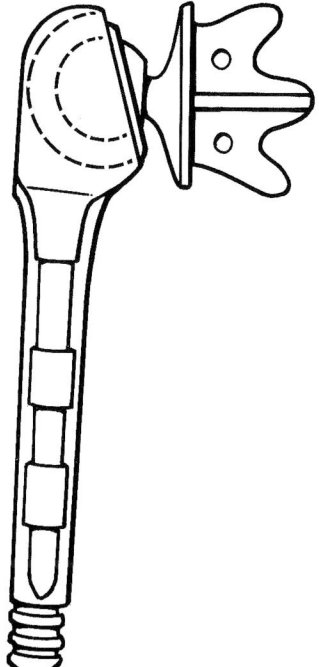 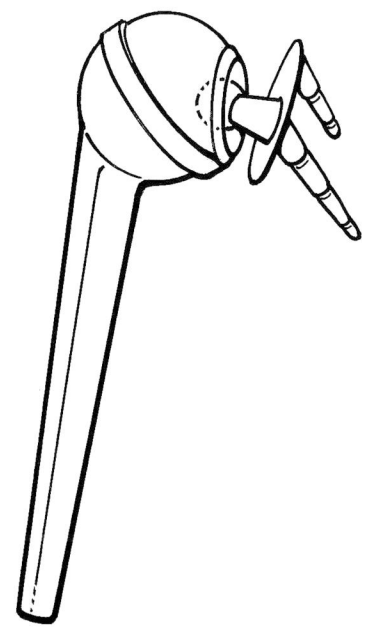

FIGURE 12
The Neer Mark III. The reverse ball and socket also allowed for rotation of the stem within the humeral component. This was a clever design; however, it did not work as well as hoped and was discontinued in 1974.

FIGURE 13
Floating Socket. This was a reverse bipolar type of design. The large head and two points of rotation theoretically allowed for greater mobility. In reality, this did not work as theorized.

important safety factor that should be designed into the appliance. Indications for this type of shoulder replacement are quite limited. This was the most popular North American constrained total shoulder arthroplasty, and it was used well into the 1990s.

The Neer Mark III was a reverse ball-and-socket design that had a clever addition of axial rotation of the humeral component within the humeral sleeve (Fig. 12). It was abandoned in 1974.

The Fenlin[38] and the Floating Socket[39] were similar designs. Both are of the large-head, reversed ball-and-socket design (Fig. 13). The Fenlin heavily invaded the glenoid vault for scapular fixation, whereas the Floating Socket used the cortical bone of the glenoid for support. The design of these appliances allowed for a greater range of motion and pain relief, but neither delivered the desired durability or return of function. The only surviving constrained appliance in Europe today, the Delta III, seems to have many of the design characteristics of these two earlier appliances. The Delta III appliance was used with promising early success by Ekelund and associates[40] as a salvage procedure for eight patients with instability and pain following failed shoulder arthroplasty.

The Kessel and Liverpool appliances both were reversed ball-and-socket protheses with captured heads.[41,42] The Kessel was uncemented and was fixed with a large single screw-post while using the strong cortical glenoid bone for support.[41] The Liverpool looked like a reversed total shoulder arthroplasty. Beddow and Elloy[42] used the small medullary canal on the lateral wing of the scapula for its cement anchor. In a report of 23 Kessel appliances inserted between 1982 and 1985, six failed and 15 of the remaining 17 achieved excellent pain relief, but active range of motion was poor[41] and it is no longer in active use. The Liverpool, which had a high failure rate, was a technically difficult appliance to insert and is no longer available.

The Tri-spherical was an ingenious design that consolidated the promising features of all other appliances into a single product.[43] The Tri-spherical was a captured ball and socket, a captured reverse ball and socket, and a tripolar, all engineered into a single total shoulder replacement (Fig. 14). The main thought behind the design was to put together an appliance that could achieve more motion than the shoulder was physiologically capable of; thus, stresses would be absorbed by the soft tissue rather than by the anchorage of the appliance to the bone. In a 1982 publication, Gristina and Webb[43] reported on 18 patients observed from 12 to 42 months after insertion of the Tri-spherical. Pain relief was dramatic in all patients, but the overall functional gain was modest at best. The main problem with the Tri-spherical, other than its general girth, was that it had a variable fulcrum, which made it difficult to maintain active function, and it is not in active use today.

The frequent problems with glenoid fixation led to the recommendation by many to avoid the use of the glenoid component when it was not possible to stabilize the arthroplasty with a func-

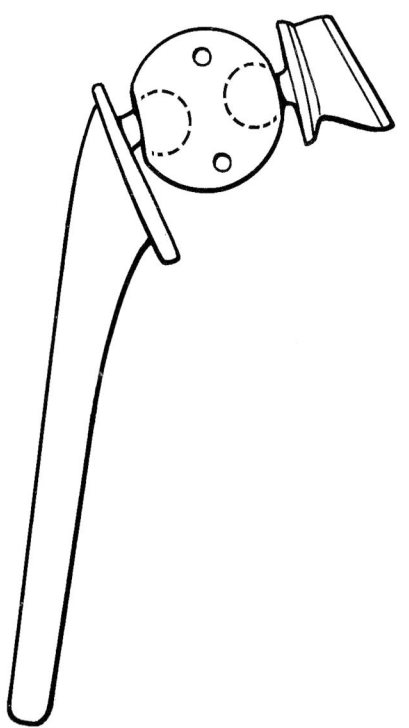

FIGURE 14
Tri-spherical. This was quite similar to Péan's initial TSA. The multiple points of mobility offered greater motion than physiologically possible in a normal shoulder, thus taking stress off of the bony fixation points. However, the variable fulcrum proved to be ineffective.

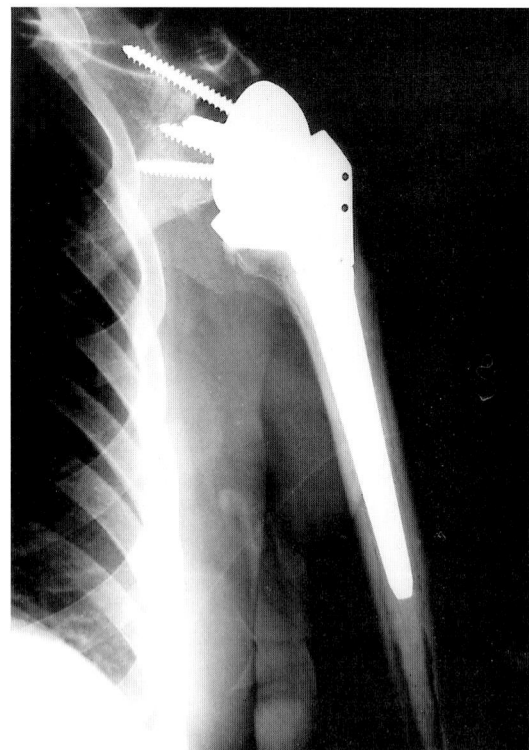

FIGURE 15
Delta III. This appears to be the sole survivor of the constrained total shoulder replacements. It remains in active use in Europe today. The design has a large head like the Fenlin and Floating Socket, surface-mounting on the glenoid like the Michael Reese, and cement-free fixation as in the Kessel. (Courtesy of Anders Ekelund, Sweden.)

tional rotator cuff. Fenlin[38] was the first to suggest the use of an oversized head to fill the soft-tissue envelope in this circumstance and thus gain stability through sheer volume. The advent of the oversized ball was a result of a difficult situation in which a patient with bilateral Charcot joints had a loosened prosthesis, bone loss of the proximal humerus, and resection of the rotator cuff. Fenlin attempted to resolve the dilemma by removing the prosthesis and replacing it with an oversized ball. Fenlin's technique can be performed with a variety of modular appliances or, as some have suggested, with an oversized bipolar (Fig. 16) appliance. The suggestion to use a bipolar appliance was a new application of an old approach suggested both by Bateman[44] and Swanson[45] for the primary treatment of painful glenohumeral arthritis. Although Fenlin does not favor the use of a bipolar, he has stayed with the oversized ball approach for 25 years. He recently reaffirmed its usefulness.[46] The consensus is, however, that this remains a difficult problem whether it is dealt with through the use of a bipolar appliance, a modular oversized appliance, or a Delta III reverse shoulder appliance.

The endeavors of the past 50 years are summarized nicely by Thomas Schenk and Joseph Iannotti:[47] "Nonconstrained prostheses have been designed to closely replicate normal bony anatomy to allow the surgeon to restore a close approximation of normal anatomic relationships. The percentage of good and excellent results and number of complications of nonconstrained shoulder arthroplasties now appear to have had little change since the earliest reports, despite an evolution of component design features and component options...constrained and semiconstrained prosthesis have rare, if any, indication for use currently...." This statement recognizes where total shoulder arthroplasty is today, but places it within the context of the efforts of dozens of physicians who attempted to improve on the earliest designs. Even the least successful of these attempts has been an overall contribution to the evolution of total shoulder arthroplasty through honest reports of success, or lack thereof, thus opening or closing potential pathways. Stated another way, we like where we are today because we have been other places and have not liked them as well.

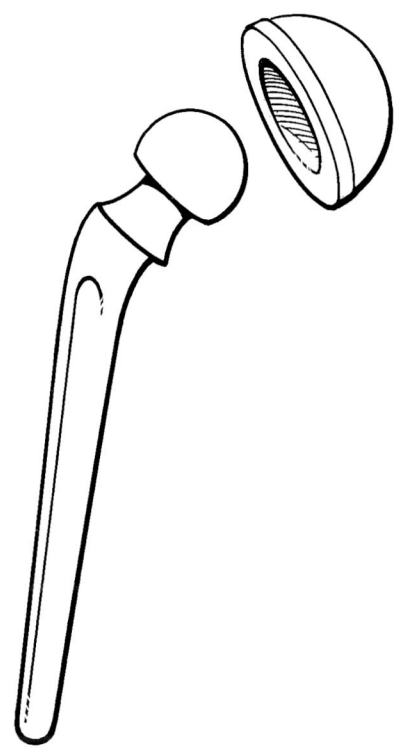

FIGURE 16
The Bipolar. As with the cup arthroplasty, this was a hip solution applied to the shoulder. This approach was originally suggested by Bateman but first implemented by Swanson.

ACKNOWLEDGMENT

Every effort has been made to be complete as well as accurate in interpreting the significance of each individual's contribution to the development of total shoulder arthroplasty; however, there may have been some misinterpretations or inadvertent exclusions, and for these, I apologize. Robert Cofield's history of total shoulder arthroplasty[1] helped enormously by mapping out where most of the information contained in this chapter could be found.

I would like to thank Jean Lundin for her assistance.

REFERENCES

1. Cofield RH: Degenerative and arthritic problems of the glenohumeral joint, in Rockwood CA Jr, Matsen FA III (eds): *The Shoulder*. Philadelphia, PA, WB Saunders, 1990, pp 678–749.

2. Péan JE: The classic: On prosthetic methods intended to repair bone fragments. *Clin Orthop* 1973;94:4–7.

3. Lugli T: Artificial shoulder by Pean (1893): The facts of an exceptional intervention and the prosthetic method. *Clin Orthop* 1978;133:215–218.

4. Gluck TH: Autoplastik: Transplantation. Implantation von Fremdkorpern. *Berl Klin Wochenschr* 1890;27:421–427.

5. Bankes MJ, Emery RJ: Pioneers of shoulder replacement: Themistocles Gluck and Jules Emile Péan. *J Shoulder Elbow Surg* 1995;4:259–262.

6. Peltier LF (ed): *Orthopedics: A History and Iconography*. San Francisco, CA, Norman Publishing, 1993.

7. Barton JR: The classic: On the treatment of anchylosis, by the formation of artificial joints. *Clin Orthop* 1984;182:4–13.

8. Ollier L (ed): *Traité Experimental et Clinique de la Regénération des os et de la Production Artificielle du Tissu Osseux*. Paris, France, Victor Masson et fils, 1867, pp 293–328.

9. Murphy JB: Arthroplasty for ankylosis joints. *Trans Am Surg Assoc* 1913;31:67–137.

10. Murphy JB: The classic: Arthroplasty for ankylosis joints. *Clin Orthop* 1986;213:4–12.

11. Baer WS: Arthroplasty with the aid of animal membrane. *Am J Orthop Surg* 1918;16:1–29, 94–115, 171–199.

12. MacAusland WR, MacAusland AR (eds): *The Mobilization of Ankylosed Joints by Arthroplasty*. Philadelphia, PA, Lea & Febiger, 1929.

13. Tillman K, Braatz D: Resection interposition arthroplasty of the shoulder in rheumatoid arthritis, in Lettin AWF, Petersson C (eds): *Rheumatoid Arthritis Surgery of the Shoulder*. Basel, Switzerland, Karger, 1989.

14. Steffee AD, Moore RW: Hemi-resurfacing arthroplasty of the shoulder. *Contemp Orthop* 1984;9:51–59.

15. Varian JPW: Abstract: Interposition silastic cup arthroplasty of the shoulder. *J Bone Joint Surg* 1980;62B:116–117.

16. Krueger FJ: A Vitallium replica arthroplasty on the shoulder: A case report of aseptic necrosis of the proximal end of the humerus. *Surgery* 1951;30:1005–1011.

17. Richard A, Judet R, Rene L: Acrylic prosthetic reconstruction of the upper end of the humerus for fracture-luxations. *J Chir* 1952;68:537–547.

18. Neer CS II: Shoulder arthroplasty: History, new designs and newer complications, in Mansat M (ed): *Les Prostheses d'Epaule*. Paris, France, Expansion Scientific Publications, 1999:1–11.

19. de Anquin CE, de Anquin CA: Prosthetic replacement in the treatment of serious fractures of the proximal humerus, in Bayley I, Kessel L (eds): *Shoulder Surgery*. Berlin, Germany, Springer-Verlag, 1982, pp 207–217.

20. Neer CS, Brown TH Jr, Mclaughlin HL: Fracture of the neck of the humerus with dislocation of the head fragment. *Am J Surg* 1953;85:252–258.

21. Neer CS II: Articular replacement for the humeral head. *J Bone Joint Surg* 1955;37A:215–228.

22. Neer CS II: Articular replacement for the humeral head. *J Bone Joint Surg* 1964;46:1607–1610.

23. Engelbrecht E, Stellbrink G: Totale Schulterendoprothese Modell "St George". *Chirurg* 1976;47:525–530.

24. Kenmore PI, MacCartee C, Vitek B: A simple shoulder replacement. *J Biomed Mater Res* 1974;8:329–330.

25. Neer CS II: Replacement arthroplasty for glenohumeral osteoarthritis. *J Bone Joint Surg* 1974;56A:1–13.

26. Zipple J: Vollstandiger: Shulterglenenkerstaz aux Kunstoff und Metall. *Biomed Tech* 1972:17:87–91.

27. Engelbrecht E, Heinert K: More than ten years' experience with unconstrained shoulder replacement, in Kölbel R, Helbig B, Blauth W (eds): *Shoulder Replacement*. Berlin, Germany, Springer-Verlag, 1987, p 85–91.

28. Amstutz HC, Thomas BJ, Kabo JM, Jinnah RH, Dorey FJ: The Dana total shoulder arthroplasty. *J Bone Joint Surg* 1988;70A:1174–1182.

29. Gristina AG, Romano RL, Kammire GC, Webb LX: Total shoulder replacement. *Orthop Clin North Am* 1987;18:445–453.

30. Mazas F, de la Caffinière JY: Total shoulder replacement by an unconstrained prosthesis: Report of 38 cases. *Rev Chir Orthop Reparatrice Appar Mot* 1982:68:161–170.

31. Franklin JL, Barrett WP, Jackins SE, Matsen FA III: Glenoid loosening in total shoulder arthroplasty: Association with rotator cuff deficiency. *J Arthroplasty* 1988;3:39–46.

32. Lettin AW, Copeland SA, Scales JT: The Stanmore total shoulder replacement. *J Bone Joint Surg* 1982:64B:47–51.

33. Cofield R: Results and complications of shoulder arthroplasty, in Morrey BF, An KN (ed): *Reconstructive Surgery of the Joints,* ed 2. New York, NY, Churchill Livingstone, 1996, pp 773–787.

34. Zippel J: Luxationssichere Schulterendoprothese Modell BME. *Z Orthop* 1975;113:454–457.

35. Post M, Haskell SS, Jablon M: Total shoulder replacement with a constrained prosthesis. *J Bone Joint Surg* 1980:62A:327–335.

36. Post M (ed): *The Shoulder: Surgical and Nonsurgical Management,* ed 2. Philadelphia, PA, Lea & Febiger, 1988, pp 221–278.

37. Post M, Jablon M, Miller H, Singh M: Constrained total shoulder joint replacement: A critical review. *Clin Orthop* 1979:144:135–150.

38. Fenlin JM Jr: Total glenohumeral joint replacement. *Orthop Clin North Am* 1975:6:565–583.

39. Buechel FF, Pappas MJ, DePalma AF: "Floating-socket" total shoulder replacement: Anatomical, biomechanical, and surgical rationale. *J Biomed Mater Res* 1978:12:89–114.

40. Ekelund A, Westerlind G, Nyberg R: Abstract. Revision of unstable shoulder arthroplasties with the inverted Delta-III prosthesis. *Acta Orthop Scand* 1997;274(suppl):90.

41. Brostrom LA, Wallensten R, Olsson E, Anderson D: The Kessel prosthesis in total shoulder arthroplasty: A five-year experience. *Clin Orthop* 1992:277:155–160.

42. Beddow FH, Elloy MA: Clinical experience with the Liverpool shoulder replacement, in Bayley I, Kessel L (eds): *Shoulder Surgery.* Berlin, Germany, Springer-Verlag, 1982, pp 164–167.

43. Gristina AG, Webb LX: The trispherical total shoulder replacement, in Bayley I, Kessel L (eds): *Shoulder Surgery.* Berlin, Germany, Springer-Verlag, 1982:153–157.

44. Bateman JE: Lesions producing the shoulder pain predominantly, in Bateman JE, Fornasier VL (eds): *The Shoulder and Neck.* Philadelphia, PA, WB Saunders, 1978, pp 242–374.

45. Swanson AB: Bipolar implant shoulder arthroplasty, in Bateman JE, Welsh RP (eds): *Surgery of the Shoulder.* Philadelphia, PA, CV Mosby, 1984, pp 211–223.

46. Fenlin JM Jr, Frieman B: Shoulder arthroplasty: Massive cuff deficiency, in Iannotti JP, Williams GR Jr (eds): *Disorders of the Shoulder: Diagnosis and Management.* Philadelphia, PA, Lippincott Williams & Wilkins, 1999, pp 559–569.

47. Schenk T, Iannotti JP: Prosthetic arthroplasty for glenohumeral arthritis with an intact or repairable rotator cuff: Indications, techniques, and results, in Iannotti JP, Williams GR Jr (eds): *Disorders of the Shoulder: Diagnosis and Management.* Philadelphia, PA, Lippincott Williams & Wilkins, 1999, pp 521–558.

INDICATIONS

JAMES M. HILL, MD

ANATOMY AND PHYSIOLOGY

The shoulder plays an important functional role in allowing an individual to position the hand in space. The function of the shoulder girdle is complex and requires the integrated motion of glenohumeral, scapulothoracic, acromioclavicular, and sternoclavicular joints. The combined function of these joints makes possible the ability to position the hand along the surface of a sphere that is centered at the shoulder. The elbow joint provides position or motion of the hand along the radius of the sphere. The combined motion of the shoulder girdle and elbow allows essential global movement, limited only by the position of the body within the sphere. Thus, restoring this motion to a severely arthritic and ankylosed shoulder joint markedly improves the function of the upper extremity.

The articular surface of the humeral head is essentially spherical, with an arc of approximately 160° covered by articular cartilage.[1] The radius of curvature is approximately 25 mm and is slightly greater in men than in women.[2,3] The average neck-shaft angle is 45° (± 5°) with a range of 30° to 55°. Retroversion of the humeral head articular surface relative to the axis of the elbow joint averages 35° but can range from 20° to 45°.[4,5] The cephalad margin of the humeral head articular surface is always superior to the top of the greater tuberosity by an average distance of 8 mm (± 3.2 mm) (Fig. 1). Maintaining this relationship has been found to correlate positively with functional outcome. Restoring the center of rotation for the humeral head relative to the axis of the humeral diaphysis has been theoretically important for avoiding eccentric forces on the glenoid. Maintaining these relationships prolongs glenoid fixation and decreases polyethylene wear.[6–8]

The glenoid is attached to the remainder of the scapular body through the glenoid neck. The glenoid has a pear-shaped articular surface with the superior-inferior dimension (average ± 3.7 mm) greater than the anterior-posterior dimension by a ratio of 1:0.7. The anterior-posterior dimension of the superior half of the glenoid articular surface is

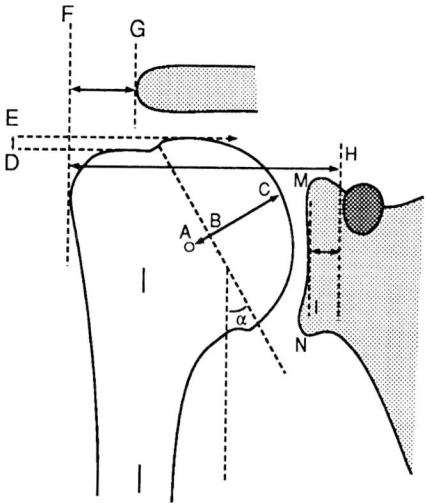

FIGURE 1
The normal glenohumeral relationships, with the humeral offset depicted by the distance F to H, the thickness of the humeral head from B to C, and the center of the humeral head at C. Note the superior position of the humeral head proximal to the greater tuberosity (D to E). (Reproduced with permission from Iannotti JP, Gabriel JP, Schneck SL, et al: The normal glenohumeral relationships: An anatomical study of one hundred and forty shoulders. J Bone Joint Surg 1992;74A:491–500.)

approximately 80% of the lower half.[2] The articular surface of the glenoid encompasses an arc of 74° (± 6°) in the anterior-posterior dimension and 96° (± 8°) in the superior-inferior dimension.[1] The glenoid articular surface radius of curvature is between 2 and 3 mm larger than that of the humeral head.[2,3] The average orientation of the glenoid surface to the axis of the scapular body, based on computed tomography (CT) studies, ranged from 2° of anteversion to 7° of retroversion.[9,10]

The lateral humeral offset is defined as the distance from the lateral base of the coracoid process to the lateral margin of the greater tuberosity.[2] Significantly decreasing this distance results in reduced level arms for the deltoid and supraspinatus, which impairs function by weakening abduction at the glenohumeral joint.[11] In addition, this may result in soft-tissue laxity and possibly joint instability. Significantly increasing the lateral humeral offset will cause excessive tension on the soft tissues. This results in over-stuffing the joint and associated loss of motion.

A variety of conditions affect the shoulder, causing progressive loss of the articular cartilage. The resultant arthritis may be accompanied by other pathologic changes such as bone loss, capsular laxity or contracture, and rotator cuff rupture. The combined effect of these processes results in pain, loss of joint motion, and perhaps loss of joint stability. Consequently, function of the shoulder joint is impaired. Several conditions cause arthritis of the glenohumeral joint, with resulting progressive pain and loss of function. Each process is associated with typical and unique alterations of the bone and soft tissues.

OSTEOARTHRITIS

Primary osteoarthritis is the most common arthritic process affecting the shoulder. Up to 60% of patients undergoing total shoulder replacement carry a diagnosis of primary osteoarthritis.[12–21] The common radiographic changes in osteoarthritis include joint space narrowing, marginal osteophyte formation, subchondral sclerosis, and cysts (Fig. 2).

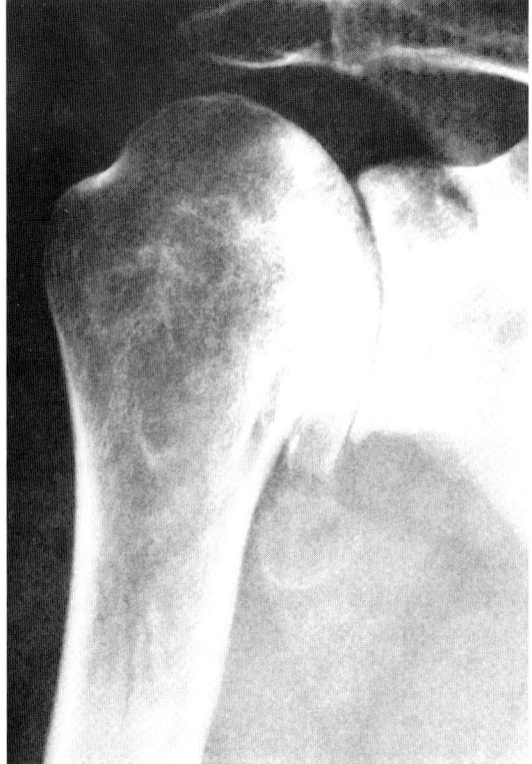

FIGURE 2
Severe osteoarthritis with large inferior osteophyte (goat's beard), loss of glenohumeral joint space, sclerotic bone formation, and periarticular cyst formation.

The specific pathologic changes were accurately described by Neer and associates.[12,19] Osteophytes are most prominent along the inferior and posterior margins of the humeral head. They often can obscure the anatomic margin of the humeral head, especially in the calcar region. In addition, they can enlarge the humeral head up to twice its normal size. This enlargement can cause capsular distention, most common in the posterior region. The glenoid surface often is eburnated with central or more commonly posterior erosion.[22] The combination of posterior capsular distention and posterior glenoid erosion can lead to posterior glenohumeral instability that may have to be addressed at total shoulder arthroplasty with either capsular reefing or glenoid bone grafting. The incidence of complete rotator cuff tears in patients with osteoarthritis is less than 10%.[14,18,19,23] There often is a contracture of the subscapularis tendon in osteoarthritis that may require release either by tendon mobilization or Z-lengthening.[12]

RHEUMATOID ARTHRITIS

Rheumatoid arthritis is the second most common diagnosis for patients undergoing total shoulder arthroplasty. Combining the data for the larger studies on unconstrained shoulder replacement, rheumatoid arthritis accounts for approximately 31% of patients undergoing this procedure.[13–21] The pathologic changes that occur with this disease process are secondary to chronic synovial inflammation and pannus formation. The synovitis and subsequent release of inflammatory mediators results in the characteristic destruction of both bone and soft tissue. The extent to which this occurs varies between patients.

Common radiographic changes in rheumatoid arthritis include osteopenia and periarticular erosions. Osteoporosis may result from steroid use or the disease process itself. Cortical thinning at the humerus, softening of the humeral cancellous bone, and marginal erosions at the humeral head may preclude press-fit fixation of the humeral component, thus necessitating cement fixation. Rheumatoid granulation tissue causes subchondral glenoid cyst formation, which typically is manifested as central or superior erosion of the glenoid articular surface (Fig. 3). The resultant joint centralization and decrease in glenoid volume may require cancellous bone grafting of these typically contained defects for adequate glenoid component support.[19,22,23]

The chronic inflammatory process in rheumatoid arthritis also weakens the soft tissues. The rotator cuff often is attenuated or frankly torn. The incidence of full-thickness rotator cuff tears varies in the literature from 8% to 42% of patients treated with shoulder arthroplasty, with the average being between 20% and 30%.[14,15,18,19,23–27] The presence of a rotator cuff tear has been shown to adversely affect the overall functional score, range of motion, and glenoid component fixation with total shoulder arthroplasty.[14,18,19,23–27]

TRAUMATIC ARTHRITIS

Arthritis secondary to chronic displaced fractures and fracture-dislocations of the glenohumeral joint accounts for up to 24% of patients treated with shoulder arthroplasty. Combining the data for the larger studies on unconstrained shoulder replacement, posttraumatic arthritis accounts for approximately 13% of patients undergoing this procedure.[13–21] This is a particularly difficult arthritic process to treat with replacement arthroplasty because it is commonly associated with contracture and scarring of the soft tissues, malunion or nonunion of the tuberosities, and possible nerve injuries. The soft-tissue contractures may prove difficult to fully release, thus impairing restoration of motion. Osteotomy and fixation of the tuberosities may delay the postoperative rehabilitation or impair rotator cuff strength. Neer and associates[19] reported axillary nerve palsy in 7 of 60 patients (12%) with posttraumatic arthritis. This injury significantly impairs motion and strength from loss of deltoid function.

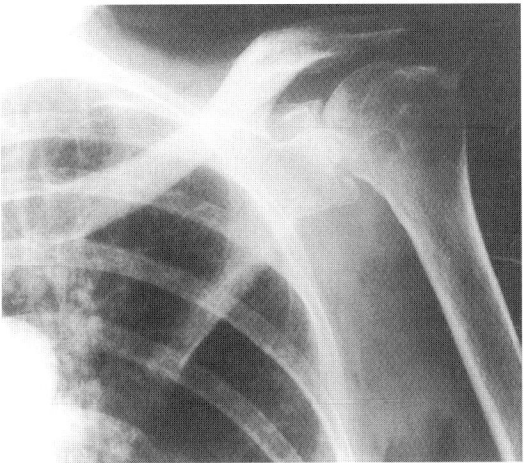

FIGURE 3
Rheumatoid arthritis with central erosion of the glenoid surface, lack of osteophyte generation, cortical thinning of the proximal humerus, and periarticular erosions.

OSTEONECROSIS

Nontraumatic osteonecrosis of the humeral head results from damage to the vascular supply in the region. The most common causes for this process include corticosteroid use, sickle cell disease, and alcoholism. However, it is not uncommon for the disease to be idiopathic. Less common causes include dysbarism, Gaucher's disease, and systemic lupus erythematosus. The incidence of osteonecrosis in patients treated with total shoulder arthroplasty is approximately 3%.[13-21] The disease process is classified most commonly using the radiographic staging system devised by Cruess[28] (Fig. 4). Stage I is documented only by scintigraphy or magnetic resonance imaging. Stage II demonstrates localized or mottled sclerosis. Stage III is represented by the presence of the "crescent" sign. Stage IV is characterized by significant collapse of the humeral head subchondral bone. Stage V disease has degenerative changes at both sides of the joint. The natural history of humeral head osteonecrosis is rather variable and often quite benign. Rutherford and Cofield[29] found that clinical progression occurred in only 2 of 11 patients with stage II or III disease. However, all five patients with stages IV or V disease demonstrated symptomatic progression over time (Fig. 5). In 17 other patients with marked symptoms, 10 were treated with humeral head replacement alone. Seven patients required total shoulder arthroplasty. However, L'Insalata and

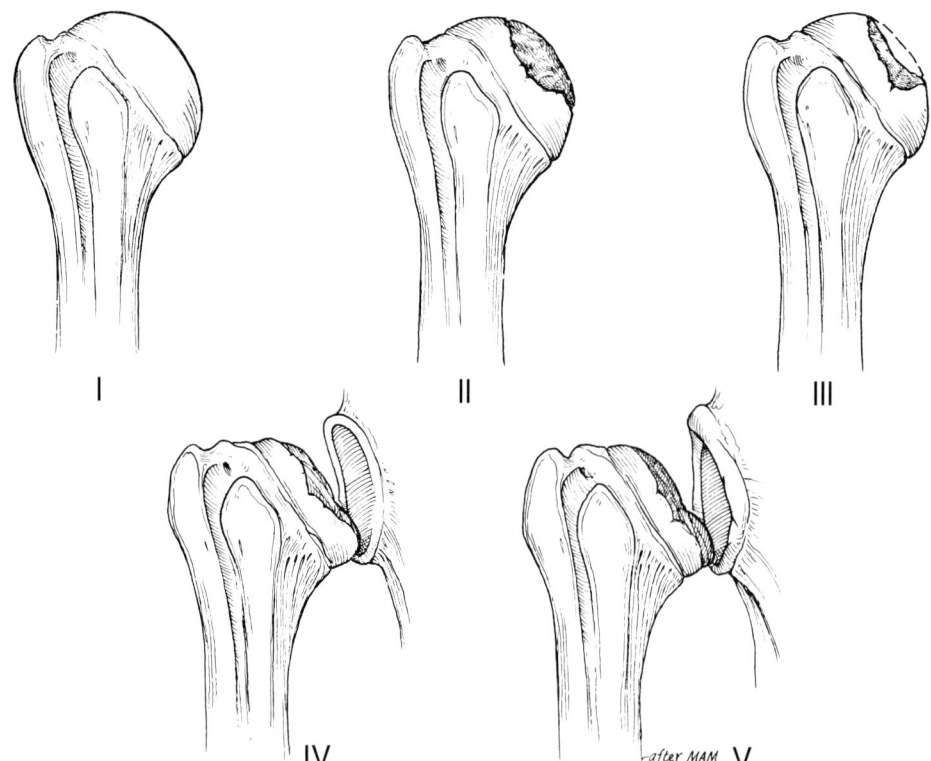

FIGURE 4
Stages of osteonecrosis of the humeral head. Stage I changes are not visible on plain radiographs, nor are they discernible on gross examination. Stage II is marked by sclerotic changes and evidence of bone remodeling, but the shape and sphericity of the humeral head are maintained. Stage III is differentiated from stage II by the presence of subchondral bone collapse or fracture, resulting in loss of humeral head sphericity. In stage IV, the humeral head has an area of collapsed articular surface; the fragment may become displaced intra-articularly. In stage V, there are osteoarthritic changes in the glenoid fossa. (Reproduced with permission from Cushner MA, Friedman RJ: Osteonecrosis of the humeral head. *J Am Acad Orthop Surg* 1997;5:339–346.)

associates[30] found symptomatic progression of the disease to severe pain and disability in 71% of 65 shoulders. Fifty-three percent of the 65 shoulders required shoulder arthroplasty.

CAPSULORRHAPHY ARTHRITIS

Neer and associates[19] described an arthropathy associated with patients who experienced recurrent dislocations and had been treated with an instability repair procedure. This condition currently is termed capsulorrhaphy arthropathy. These patients accounted for 10% of their patient population undergoing total shoulder arthroplasty. This condition is believed to result from excessive soft-tissue tension on the side of dislocation producing a fixed subluxation of the humeral head in the opposite direction. Glenoid erosion is more severe than in primary osteoarthritis, sometimes necessitating peripheral corticocancellous bone grafting. It is recommended to obtain a CT scan prior to surgery to evaluate the glenoid (Fig. 6). In addition, the iatrogenic soft-tissue contracture requires release to restore joint balance and mobility.

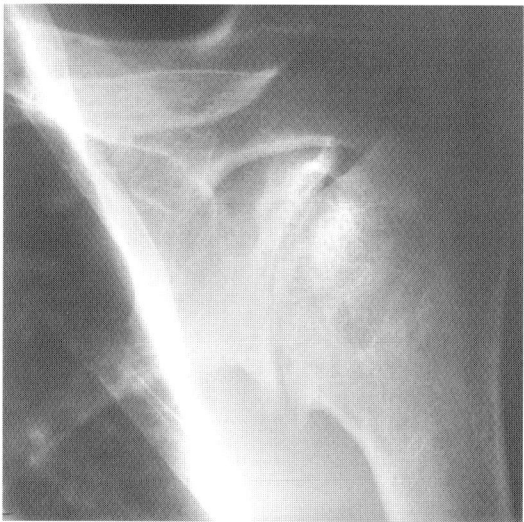

FIGURE 5
Anteroposterior radiograph of the left shoulder of a 27-year-old man with stage V osteonecrosis. (Reproduced with permission from Cushner MA, Friedman RJ: Osteonecrosis of the humeral head. J Am Acad Orthop Surg 1997;5:339–346.)

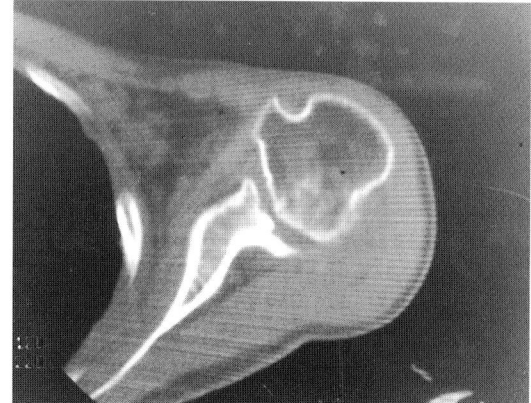

FIGURE 6
Computed tomography scan revealing large posterior osteophyte with subluxated humeral head.

ROTATOR CUFF ARTHROPATHY

A distinct form of osteoarthritis, associated with a chronic massive tear of the rotator cuff, was first described by Neer and associates[31] in 1983. This condition was termed cuff tear arthropathy and is characterized by massive rotator cuff tear, glenohumeral arthritis, and glenohumeral instability. The instability is manifested as proximal migration of the humerus relative to the glenoid, resulting in erosion of the caudal surface of the acromion and eburnation of the greater tuberosity (Fig. 7). Premature glenoid component loosening has been associated with rotator cuff tears.[14,18,32] Early attempts at "hooding" the glenoid along the superior margin failed to improve functional results. Irreparable tears of the rotator cuff generally are considered a relative contraindication for glenoid resurfacing. A more satisfactory long-term result in cuff tear arthropathy may be obtained with isolated humeral head replacement.

MANAGEMENT

Several treatment options are available for the patient with glenohumeral arthritis. The mainstay of treatment remains medical management with the use of nonsteroidal anti-inflammatory medications. Nutritional supplementation with glu-

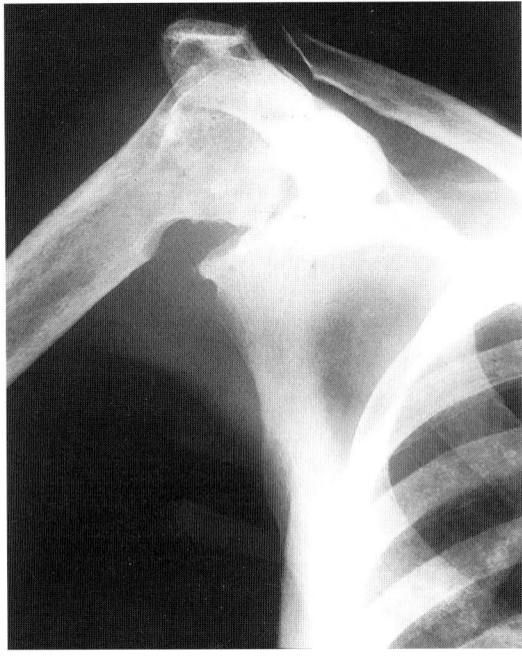

FIGURE 7
Anteroposterior radiograph shows rotator cuff-tear arthropathy in the right shoulder of a 77-year-old man. The shoulder is in maximum active abduction. In addition to humeral head collapse, findings include periarticular osteopenia, reduced acromiohumeral distance, and erosions of the glenoid, acromion, and acromioclavicular joint. (Reproduced with permission from Zeman CA, Arcand MA, Cantrell JS, Skedros JG, Burkhead WZ Jr: The rotator cuff-deficient arthritic shoulder: Diagnosis and surgical management. *J Am Acad Orthop Surg* 1998;6:337–348.)

cosamine and chondroitin sulfate may also provide some symptomatic control. Patients with more severe forms of inflammatory arthropathy may benefit from oral steroids or other immunosupressive medications such as methotrexate. Physical therapy can help maintain motion and strength. Intra-articular corticosteroid injections often provide significant but temporary relief. However, the use of these injections should be limited due to known deleterious effects on soft tissues and residual cartilage.

Once conservative management fails to adequately control symptoms, surgical options can be considered. Shoulder synovectomy has been used in an attempt to control pain for the rheumatoid disease. In general, this is most appropriate for patients who have maintained the articular cartilage. Although pain relief may be adequate, motion is not expected to improve appreciably. Resection arthroplasty of the shoulder is predominately of historical interest. It has a potential application in the treatment of severe septic arthritis resulting in osteomyelitis of the humeral head or glenoid. It also may be required to treat a shoulder implant that failed because of infection or severe bone loss. However, pain relief is unpredictable with this procedure. Approximately 50% to 65% of patients will experience satisfactory pain relief. The resultant joint instability dictates extremely poor motion, strength, and function. Active abduction is less than 90°.[33]

Arthrodesis of the glenohumeral joint was the most reliable form of treatment for arthritic conditions of the shoulder prior to resurfacing arthroplasty (Fig. 8). Pain relief with this procedure is considered acceptable in approximately 75% of patients.[34] However, significant functional deficits remain, with most patients unable to perform work at or above shoulder level. Functions requiring rotational motions at the shoulder were markedly limited.[35] Currently, the major indications for arthrodesis of the shoulder include combined paralysis of the deltoid and rotator cuff, uncontrolled joint instability, and infection. Some authors consider young patients with heavy lifting

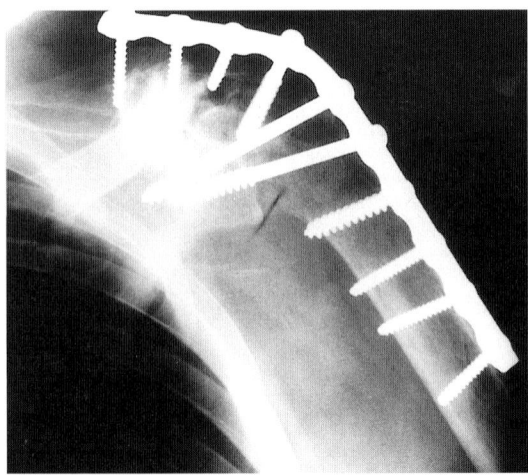

FIGURE 8
Arthrodesis of the glenohumeral joint.

demands a reasonable candidate for fusion.[36]

The primary indication for performing humeral head replacement or total shoulder arthroplasty is pain relief. In general, this procedure should be considered the treatment of choice for active patients with disabling pain that is unresponsive to conservative treatment. The patient should be considered a satisfactory surgical risk with a reasonable life expectancy. Postoperatively, 71% to 96% of all patients experience mild to no pain.[13–15,17,18,20,21,23,24,26,36–39]

A secondary goal of endoprosthetic replacement is improved motion and function. Considering all diagnostic categories, elevation improved between 27° and 50°, with external rotation increasing between 16° and 43°.[13,15,17,38,40] Functional results were considered good to excellent in 64% to 89% of patients.[13,14,19,23–25] Overall, results were believed to correlate with the diagnostic category. Osteonecrosis and osteoarthritis were shown to demonstrate better motion and functional gains relative to rheumatoid arthritis and posttraumatic arthritis.[19,23,37] However, others have not seen this correlation.[18,36] The presence of a rotator cuff tear has consistently been shown to have a negative influence on the results regarding motion and function.[13,14,18,19,24,26] Shoulder replacement arthroplasty is contraindicated in chronic infections of the joint, combined paralysis of the deltoid and rotator cuff, and uncontrolled instability of the joint. A relative contraindication is a neuropathic joint.

SUMMARY

The indications for humeral head replacement versus total shoulder arthroplasty remain controversial. Resurfacing of the glenoid was found to provide better pain relief and functional improvement relative to isolated humeral head replacement.[36,38,40] The incidence of glenoid component loosening is significantly greater than for the humeral component. In 1993, Brems[41] reviewed all literature documenting glenoid component fixation. Thirty-eight percent of all total shoulder arthroplasties demonstrated lucent lines surrounding the glenoid component fixation. Most of these lines were present on initial postoperative radiographs and failed to progress on long-term follow-up. However, 3% of all total shoulder arthroplasties require revision for symptomatic glenoid component loosening. The presence of an irreparable rotator cuff tear has been correlated with early glenoid component loosening by the "rocking horse" effect.[32] Thus, humeral head replacement is the treatment of choice for cuff arthropathy or irreparable rotator cuff tears, inadequate glenoid volume for component support and fixation, and uncorrected glenohumeral instability.

REFERENCES

1. Jobe CM, Iannotti JP: Limits imposed on glenohumeral motion by joint geometry. *J Shoulder Elbow Surg* 1995;4:281–285.

2. Iannotti JP, Gabriel JP, Schneck SL, Evans BG, Misra S: The normal glenohumeral relationships. *J Bone Joint Surg* 1992;74A:491–500.

3. Soslowsky LJ, Flatow EL, Bigliani LU, Mow VC: Articular geometry of the glenohumeral joint. *Clin Orthop* 1992;285:181–190.

4. Kronberg M, Brostrom LA, Soderlund V: Retroversion of the humeral head in the normal shoulder and its relationship to the normal range of motion. *Clin Orthop* 1990;253:13–117.

5. Pearl ML, Volk AG: Retroversion of the proximal humerus in relationship to prosthetic replacement arthroplasty. *J Shoulder Elbow Surg* 1995;4:286–289.

6. Ballmer FT, Sidles JA, Lippitt SB, Matsen FA: Humeral head prosthetic arthroplasty: Surgically relevant geometric considerations. *J Shoulder Elbow Surg* 1993;2:296–304.

7. Boileau P, Walch G: The three-dimensional geometry of the proximal humerus: Implications for surgical technique and prosthetic design. *J Bone Joint Surg* 1997;79B:857–965.

8. Pearl ML, Kurutz S: Geometric analysis of commonly used prosthetic systems for proximal humeral replacement. *J Bone Joint Surg* 1999;81A:660–671.

9. Friedman RJ, Hawthorne KB, Genez BM: The use of computerized tomography in the mea-

surement of glenoid version. *J Bone Joint Surg* 1992;74A:1032–1037.

10. Randelli M, Gambrioli PL: Glenohumeral osteometry by computerized tomography in normal and unstable shoulders. *Clin Orthop* 1986;208:151–156.

11. Rietveld ABM, Daanen HAM, Rozing PM, Oberman WR: The lever arm in glenohumeral abduction after hemiarthroplasty. *J Bone Joint Surg* 1988;70B:561–565.

12. Neer CS II: Replacement arthroplasty for glenohumeral osteoarthritis. *J Bone Joint Surg* 1974;56A:1–13.

13. Amstutz HC, Thomas BJ, Kabo JM, Jinnah RH, Dorey FJ: The Dana total shoulder arthroplasty. *J Bone Joint Surg* 1988;70A:1174–1182.

14. Barrett WP, Franklin JL, Jackins SE, Wyss CR, Matsen FA III: Total shoulder arthroplasty. *J Bone Joint Surg* 1987;69A:865–872.

15. Brenner BC, Ferlic DC, Clayton ML, Dennis DA: Survivorship of unconstrained total shoulder arthroplasty. *J Bone Joint Surg* 1989;71A:1289–1296.

16. Cofield RH, Edgerton BC: Total shoulder arthroplasty: Complications and revision surgery, in Greene WB (ed): *Instructional Course Lectures XXXIX.* Park Ridge, IL, American Academy of Orthopaedic Surgeons, 1990, pp 449–462.

17. Gristina AG, Romano RL, Kammire GC, Webb LX: Total shoulder replacement. *Orthop Clin North Am* 1987;18:445–453.

18. Hawkins RJ, Bell RH, Jallay B: Total shoulder arthroplasty. *Clin Orthop* 1989;242:188–194.

19. Neer CS II, Watson KC, Stanton FJ: Recent experience in total shoulder replacement. *J Bone Joint Surg* 1982;64A:319–337.

20. Roper BA, Paterson JM, Day WH: The Roper-Day total shoulder replacement. *J Bone Joint Surg* 1990;72B:694–697.

21. Weiss AP, Adams MA, Moore JR, Weiland AJ: Unconstrained shoulder arthroplasty: A five-year average follow-up study. *Clin Orthop* 1990;257:86–90.

22. Neer CS II, Morrison DS: Glenoid bone-grafting in total shoulder arthroplasty. *J Bone Joint Surg* 1988;70A:1154–1162.

23. Cofield RH: Total shoulder arthroplasty with the Neer prosthesis. *J Bone Joint Surg* 1984;66A:899–906.

24. Figgie HE III, Inglis AE, Goldberg VM, Ranawat CS, Figgie MP, Wile JM: An analysis of factors affecting the long-term results of total shoulder arthroplasty in inflammatory arthritis. *J. Arthroplasty* 1988;3:123–130.

25. Kelly IG, Foster RS, Fisher WD: Neer total shoulder replacement in rheumatoid arthritis. *J Bone Joint Surg* 1987;69B:723–726.

26. McCoy SR, Warren RF, Bade HA III, Ranawat CS, Inglis AE: Total shoulder arthroplasty in rheumatoid arthritis. *J Arthroplasty* 1989;4:105–113.

27. Thomas BJ, Amstutz HC, Cracchiolo A: Shoulder arthroplasty for rheumatoid arthritis. *Clin Orthop* 1991;265:125–128.

28. Cruess RL: Experience with steroid-induced avascular necrosis of the shoulder and etiologic considerations regarding osteonecrosis of the hip. *Clin Orthop* 1978;130:86–93.

29. Rutherford CS, Cofield RH: Osteonecrosis of the shoulder. *Orthop Trans* 1987;11:239.

30. L'Insalata JC, Pagnani MJ, Warren RF, Dines DM: Humeral head osteonecrosis: Clinical course and radiographic predictors of outcome. *J Shoulder Elbow Surg* 1996;5:355–361.

31. Neer CS II, Craig EV, Fukuda H: Cuff-tear arthropathy. *J Bone Joint Surg* 1983;65A:1232–1244.

32. Franklin JL, Barrett WP, Jackins SE, Matsen FA III: Glenoid loosening in total shoulder arthroplasty: Association with rotator cuff deficiency. *J Arthroplasty* 1988;3:39–46.

33. Cofield RH: Shoulder arthrodesis and resection arthroplasty, in Stauffers ES (ed): American Academy of Orthopaedic Surgeons *Instructional Course Lectures XXXIV.* St Louis, MO, CV Mosby, 1985, pp 268–277.

34. Cofield RH, Briggs BT: Glenohumeral arthrodesis: Operative and long-term functional results. *J Bone Joint Surg* 1979;61A:668–677.

35. Hawkins RJ, Neer CS II: A functional analysis of shoulder fusions. *Clin Orthop* 1987;223:65–76.

36. Bell SN, Gschwend N: Clinical experience with total arthroplasty and hemiarthroplasty of the shoulder using the Neer prosthesis. *Int Orthop* 1986;10:217–222.

37. Bade HA III, Warren RF, Ranawat CS, Inglis AE: Long term results of Neer total shoulder replacement, in Bateman JE, Welsh RP (eds): *Surgery of the Shoulder*. Philadelphia, PA, BC Decker, 1984, pp 294–302.

38. Clayton ML, Ferlic DC, Jeffers PD: Prosthetic arthroplasties of the shoulder. *Clin Orthop* 1982; 164:184–191.

39. Wilde AH, Borden LS, Brems JJ: Experience with the Neer total shoulder replacement, in Bateman JE, Welsh RP (eds): *Surgery of the Shoulder*. Philadelphia, PA, BC Decker, 1984, pp 224–228.

40. Boyd AD Jr, Thomas WH, Scott RD, Sledge CB, Thornhill TS: Total shoulder arthroplasty versus hemiarthroplasty: Indications for glenoid resurfacing. *J Arthroplasty* 1990;5:329–336.

41. Brems J: The glenoid component in total shoulder arthroplasty. *J Shoulder Elbow Surg* 1993;2: 47–54.

SURGICAL TECHNIQUE AND RESULTS

JULIAN S. ARROYO, MD

INTRODUCTION

The indications for shoulder arthroplasty are similar to those for arthroplasty of other joints. Patients with glenohumeral arthritis who have failed conservative nonsurgical measures and continue to have pain and limited function can be considered candidates for shoulder replacement surgery.

RADIOGRAPHS

Good preoperative radiographs are necessary to allow for templating and surgical planning. Five views of the shoulder should be obtained. These include anteroposterior (AP) views in neutral, internal, and external rotation; a supraspinatus outlet or scapular "Y" view; and an axillary view. The AP views will show inferior osteophytes, humeral wear, and canal diameter. The axillary view is extremely important in that it will allow observation of glenoid wear (typically posteriorly) and version of the glenoid. The outlet view demonstrates any proximal humeral migration, giving an indication of rotator cuff integrity (Fig. 1).

SURGICAL TECHNIQUE

ANESTHESIA AND POSITIONING

Either regional or general anesthesia, or a combination of the two can be used. The advantage of

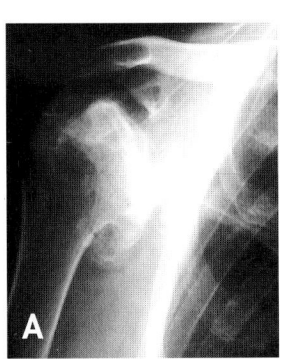
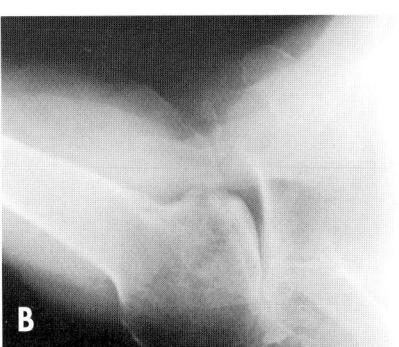
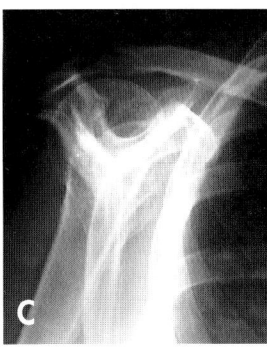

FIGURE 1
A, Anteroposterior radiograph of a 74-year-old man with osteoarthritis. Note the wear of the glenohumeral joint and the extremely large inferior osteophyte. **B,** Axillary view of the same patient. There is significant posterior wear of the joint as well as a locking posterior osteophyte that was clinically limiting external rotation. This view is extremely important for intraoperative planning. To dislocate the head, the osteophyte has to be elevated over the posterior rim of the glenoid. Without the axillary view, forced external rotation could result in a humerus fracture. This view also shows the amount of posterior translation of the joint, which may result in posterior instability of a prosthesis. **C,** Outlet view of a patient with a massive rotator cuff tear and cuff tear arthropathy. Note the proximal humeral migration and articulation of the superior aspect of the humeral head and the undersurface of the acromion. This patient would not be a good candidate for a total shoulder arthroplasty because of the incompetent rotator cuff.

an interscalene regional block is that it provides excellent muscle relaxation, facilitating the surgical exposure.[1] It also requires little or no general anesthetic agents, and the postoperative morbidity related to general anesthetic agents is reduced.[2] However, regional anesthesia can be more time consuming and is highly dependent on the experience of the anesthesiologist.

Patients are placed in the beach chair position, sitting up approximately 45°, with a small bolster under the scapula on the side undergoing surgery (Fig. 2). The patient needs to be far enough over on the table to allow for the shoulder and arm to be hyperextended. This hyperextension will be necessary during the procedure for dislocating the humerus as well as resurfacing the glenoid.

A headrest will help hold the neck in a neutral position and provide greater access to the shoulder. Securing the head to the headrest will keep the patient from sliding off of the table during the procedure. Care must be taken by the anesthesiologist to periodically inspect the position of the patient and the patient's neck to ensure that the neck remains in a neutral position. If the patient slides over, the neck can be hyperextended, placing increased traction on the brachial plexus.

SURGICAL APPROACH

A deltopectoral approach is used. A 10-cm incision is made from the clavicle, over the coracoid, to the insertion of the deltoid (Fig. 3). The cephalic vein is identified and used as the landmark for the deltopectoral interval. The vein should be dissected free and taken medially with the pectoralis. There are a number of perforators coming from the deltoid into the cephalic vein. These can be coagulated. Proximally there is a deep crossover vein that will need to be coagulated to allow for maximum exposure.

Next, any adhesions or bursa on the undersurface of the deltoid are freed from the proximal

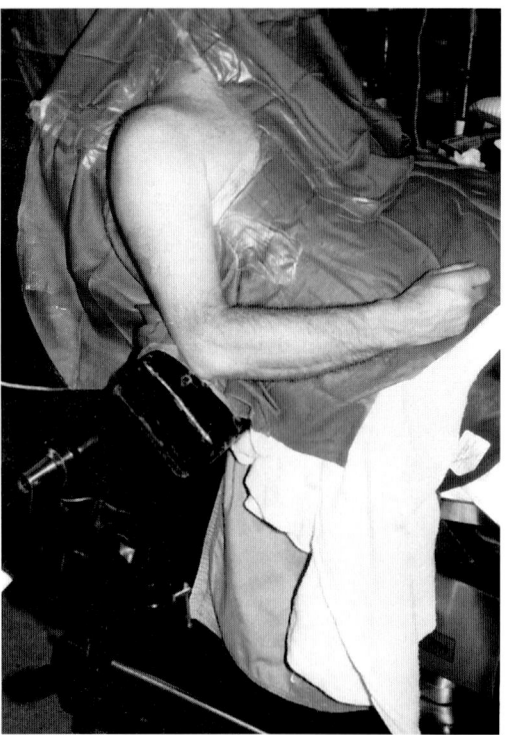

FIGURE 2
Beach chair position for total shoulder arthroplasty. The patient is flexed approximately 30° at the hips, 45° at the knees, and sat up approximately 45°. The patient is positioned laterally on the table with a small bolster under the scapula so the entire shoulder girdle and arm can be prepped freely. The arm must be able to be extended without interference from the operating table.

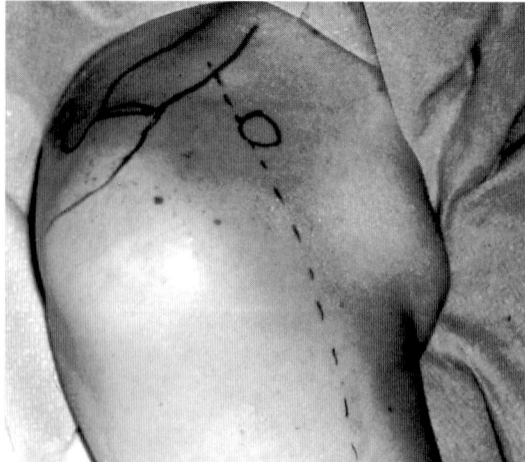

FIGURE 3
Skin incision for a deltopectoral approach. The incision begins over the clavicle and is carried over the coracoid to the insertion of the deltoid on the humerus. Note the entire shoulder girdle is prepped and exposed.

humerus and subacromial space. This is done by blunt, finger dissection, working completely around posteriorly on the humerus. Care must be taken not to tear the anterior humeral circumflex artery because it travels with the axillary nerve on the undersurface of the deltoid. Similarly, the strap muscles are carefully freed from any bursal tissue between them and the subscapularis.

The rotator cuff should be inspected for any tears. If there is a tear it will need to be repaired before final closure. Repair is done in typical fashion, with mobilization of the cuff and preparation of the tuberosity. Once the humeral head has been osteotomized, bone tunnels and sutures can be placed in the greater tuberosity for eventual repair of the rotator cuff after the humeral head is put into place.

At this point, the axillary nerve should be identified. It can be felt beneath the strap muscles medially, near the inferior margin of the subscapularis muscle. The "tug test"[3] is an excellent way to identify the nerve if it is not readily felt. One finger is placed first on the undersurface of the coracoid, and then with a sweeping motion, the finger is brought down to the bottom of the subscapularis, beneath the strap muscles (Fig. 4). The surgeon's other hand is then placed laterally, under the anterior aspect of the deltoid, finding the terminal end of the axillary nerve. The terminal end is then gently tensioned or tugged. This should cause a tugging sensation on the finger that is beneath the strap muscles, identifying the axillary nerve medially. Not uncommonly, the nerve is scarred or under tension from inferior humeral osteophytes, and only a small excursion of the nerve can be felt. The axillary nerve needs to be periodically identified and protected throughout the procedure.

With the axillary nerve identified, it is now safe to take down the subscapularis. The subscapularis tendon is incised just medial to the bicipital groove (Fig. 5), starting at the rotator interval

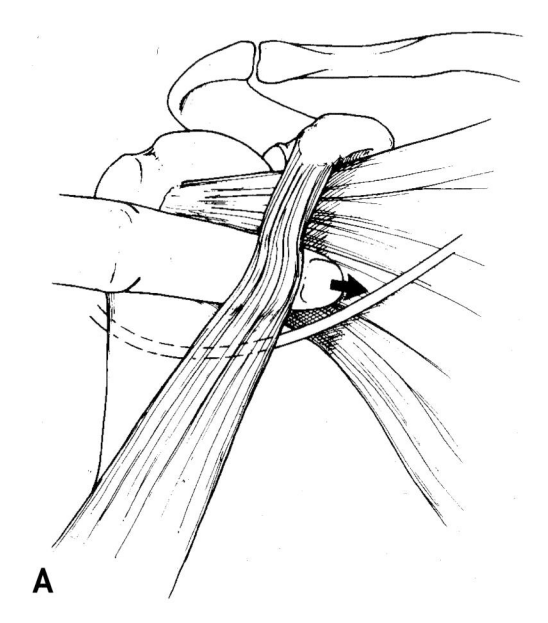

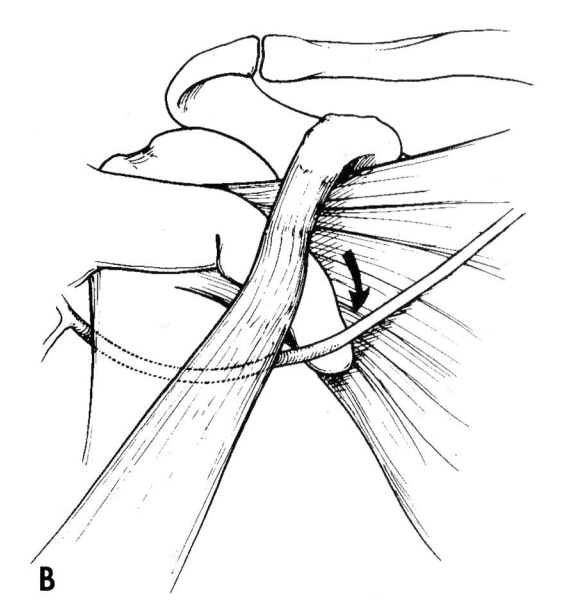

FIGURE 4
The "tug test" is used to help identify the location of the axillary nerve. **A,** The index finger is passed directly medially over the subscapularis and under the coracoid and strap muscles. **B,** The finger is then rotated down, and the axillary nerve will generally be palpable under the tip of the finger. The surgeon's other hand can be placed under the deltoid, palpating and tugging the terminal portion of the axillary nerve. This will result in a pulling or tugging of the axillary nerve medially. (Reproduced with permission from Flatow EL, Bigliani LU: Tips of the trade: Locating and protecting the axillary nerve in shoulder surgery. The tug test. *Orthop Rev* 1992;21:503–505.)

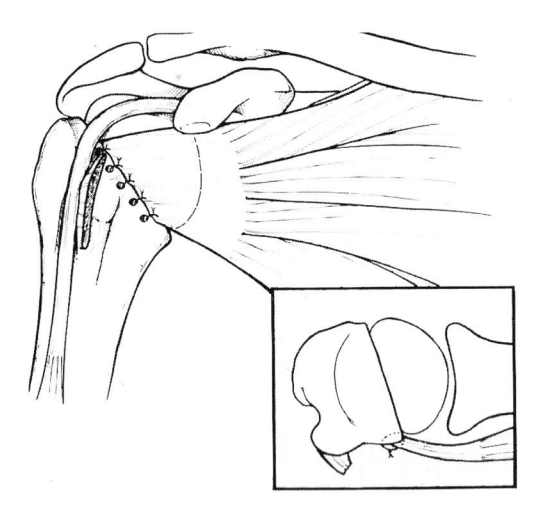

FIGURE 5
To gain maximum length of the subscapularis, it is taken down just medial to the bicipital groove, off the lesser tuberosity. After the prosthesis has been put in place and the soft tissues have been released and balanced, the subscapularis is repaired back to the lesser tuberosity in a medial position, gaining length of the tendon to maximize postoperative external rotation. (Reproduced with permission from Bigliani LU, Weinstein DM, Glasgow MT, Pollach RG, Flatow EL: Glenohumeral arthroplasty for arthritis after instability surgery. *J Shoulder Elbow Surg* 1995;4:87–94.)

proximally and going distally the entire length of the tendon. The arm is externally rotated and the subscapularis tendon and capsule are released from the anterior aspect of the humerus as one layer. Tag sutures are placed to assist in mobilization of the tendon and muscle.

Inferiorly, the capsule is often adherent beneath large osteophytes from the proximal humerus. Care must be taken while releasing this capsule because the axillary nerve passes near to this area and on occasion also will travel between the osteophytes and the humeral shaft. The capsular release should be done subperiosteally to minimize risk to the axillary nerve. Also with continued external rotation of the arm, the capsule will safely tear from the humerus. It is extremely important to release the inferior capsule to about the 8 o'clock position to later be able to translate the humeral head posteriorly and get sufficient exposure of the glenoid.

HUMERAL PREPARATION

Following the capsular release, the humeral head can be dislocated and brought anteriorly by externally rotating and extending the arm. To make an accurate humeral head cut, the peripheral osteophytes are removed with a rongeur, revealing the margin of the anatomic neck and the head (Fig. 6). The humeral head osteotomy is performed typically at 35° of retroversion, but may range between 20° and 45° of retroversion. The correct height and version are extremely important in obtaining proper soft-tissue balancing. The height of the cut is dictated by the rotator cuff insertion. The osteotomy should be made just proximal to the cuff insertion. Care must be taken not to cut in excess retroversion or the posterior insertion of the rotator cuff may be damaged or detached.

The version may be assessed either with an intramedullary guide or by positioning the arm. The arm can be held in 35° of external rotation and then an oscillating saw can be used to cut the head from directly anterior to posterior. Using this technique, it may be difficult to see the entire cuff insertion (particularly posteriorly), and it may be damaged during the osteotomy. Preferably, the arm is held in 90° of external rotation with the humeral head dislocated. This should expose the entire humeral head and allow observation of the rotator cuff insertion. The saw is then held at 35° of retroversion relative to the forearm (or 55° from the trunk of the patient), and the cut can be made safely.

The humeral shaft is then reamed and broached according to the implant system being used. The entry point for the reamers should be lateral in the head and approximately 1 cm posterior to the bicipital groove. This should centralize the body and stem of the prosthesis and provide adequate offset of the humerus.

A trial reduction at this point will allow assessment of the version, the height of the cut, and the degree of soft-tissue contracture. The prosthetic humeral head size is selected initially based on the resected head, matching the height of the resected head to a trial head. During the trial reduction, the head should lie slightly above the

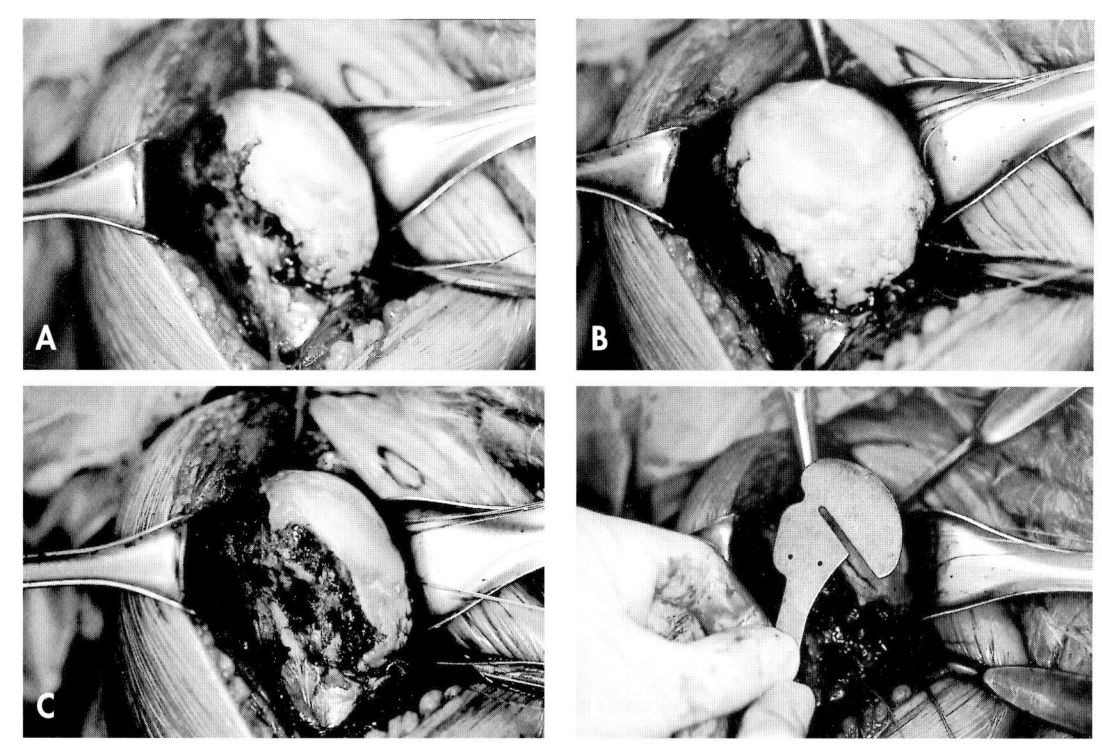

FIGURE 6
A, Peripheral osteophytes obscure the anatomic neck of the humerus. **B**, With the arm externally rotated, a large inferior osteophyte is brought into view as well as the posterior aspect of the rotator cuff (not shown here). **C**, Removing the peripheral osteophytes will reveal the anatomic neck and allow for a more accurate osteotomy of the humeral head. **D**, An external cutting guide is used to determine the inclination of the humeral osteotomy.

greater tuberosity and not excessively tent the cuff. Head selection must balance the appropriate height and offset. Final selection will be made after glenoid preparation and soft-tissue releases.

GLENOID IMPLANTATION

A humeral head retractor can be used to displace the humerus posteriorly (Fig. 7, *A*). If exposure is difficult, a more extensive subperiosteal capsular release from the humeral neck may be necessary. Anteriorly, the capsule is resected from the medial portion of the undersurface of the subscapularis and glenoid neck. A Bankart retractor can then safely be placed on the posterior glenoid neck.

The glenoid is inspected for wear and bone defects. If a glenoid component is going to be implanted, then any remaining cartilage on the surface is removed. Typically, there is posterior erosion of the glenoid, and the anterior rim of the glenoid needs to be lowered to reestablish the correct version (Fig. 8). This can be done by eccentrical reaming or with a high-speed burr. With most systems, a glenoid reamer is available. However, this may be difficult to use in a tight joint, in which case the high-speed burr can be used to contour the glenoid surface. Regardless of which technique is used, reaming should not go beyond the subchondral bone as the glenoid component needs to be supported by the intact subchondral plate.

Glenoid components will have either a keel or pegs for fixation into the glenoid vault. Whichever type is used, the component should be centered under the base of the coracoid. Positioning here will reduce the risk of glenoid neck perforation during preparation for the keel or pegs. If there is significant posterior rim wear

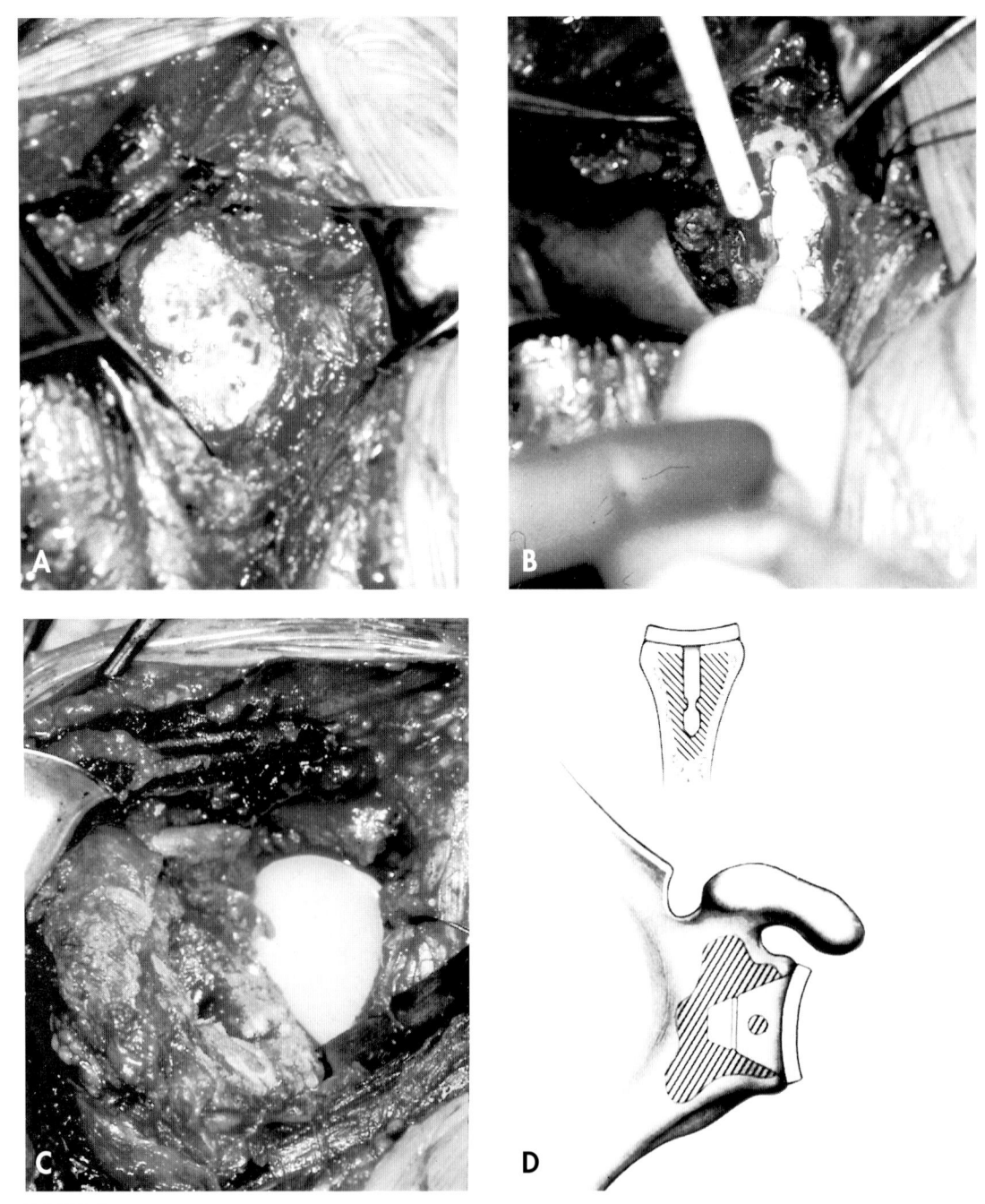

FIGURE 7
Glenoid preparation with exposure and cementing of component. **A,** Adequate glenoid exposure is obtained by a capsular release from the humeral shaft and the use of a humeral head retractor. A second retractor or a Bankart retractor is placed medially to increase the exposure. **B,** Cement is placed only in the trough and not on the subchondral bone. Cement on the subchondral bone may beak free, and support for the glenoid implant will be lost. This increases the likelihood of component loosening or breakage. **C,** The cemented component in position. **D,** Proper cementing technique will pressurize the cement into the intramedullary canal of the scapula (bottom). The component must sit flush on the subchondral bone without cement interposed (top).

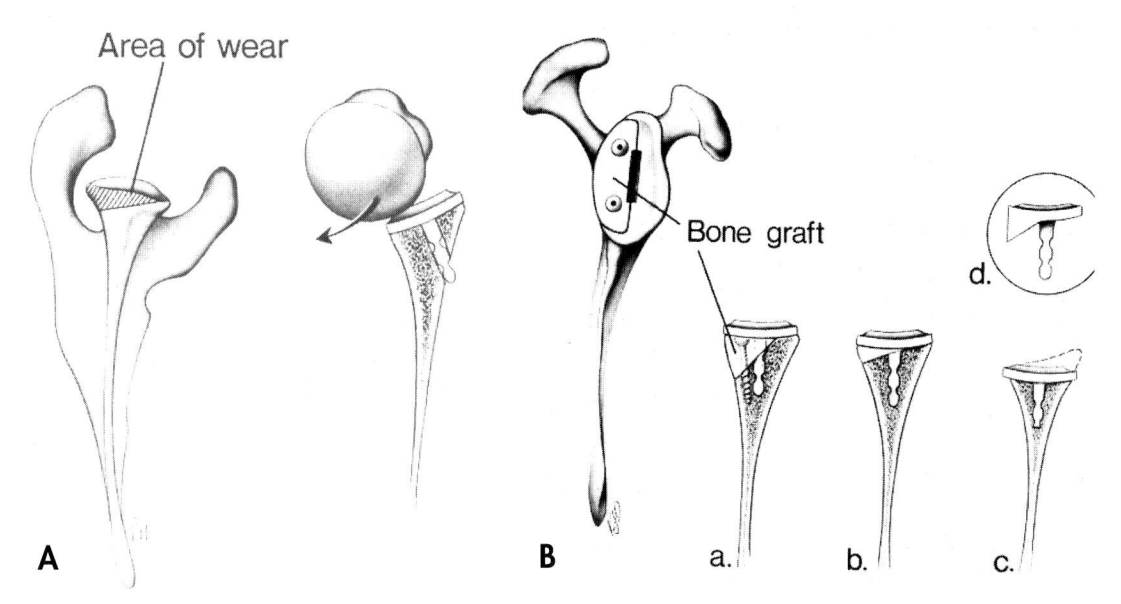

FIGURE 8
The problem and solution for uneven wear and erosion of the glenoid. **A,** If the glenoid component is cemented on the subchondral bone without correction for the wear, the anchoring device will perforate out the medullary canal. Furthermore, the tilt and loss of height make the implant unstable. **B,** The asymmetric wear of the glenoid can be corrected by bone grafting for severe cases, as shown in a. A piece of the humeral head is secured to the scapula with 4.0-mm AO navicular screws. Building up the low side with acrylic cement, as in b, or lowering the high side, as in c may offset lesser erosion. Cement is not used to correct for wear because of fear of the cement breaking loose and possible component fracture. Custom glenoid components with a thick side, shown in d, have also been developed. (Reproduced with permission from Neer CS II, Watson KC, Stanton EJ: Recent experience in total shoulder replacement. *J Bone Joint Surg* 1982;64A:319–337.)

and the anterior rim has not been lowered, then the component will sit excessively retroverted and anterior glenoid neck perforation is likely to occur (Fig. 8, *A*). Conversely, if exposure is difficult, or the anterior rim has not been lowered, there is a tendency to slot the glenoid anteriorly and perforate posteriorly.

For a keeled prosthesis, a combination of a high-speed burr and curettes are used to create the trough and avoid neck penetration. If the neck is perforated, cancellous bone from the resected head can be impacted into the defect before cementing. This will prevent cement extrusion and possible heat injury to the suprascapular nerve.

To provide secure fixation and reduce the risk of loosening, the glenoid components must sit securely against the subchondral bone of the glenoid without any rocking. Cement cannot be used to adjust for poor seating of the glenoid component.

Although press-fit and bony-ingrowth glenoid components have been developed, there is concern for higher failure rates caused by the metal backing resulting in a stiffer prosthesis with thinner polyethylene.[4] Secure cement fixation of an all-polyethylene glenoid component is recommended. To date, an effective cement pressurization system for the glenoid has not been designed. Therefore, manual pressurization is required. Whether using keeled or pegged fixation, the glenoid vault needs to be prepared for cementing. Pulse lavage is used to remove debris and blood. Hemostasis can be obtained by packing an epinephrine- or thrombin-soaked sponge into the trough or peg holes. An effective way to pressurize the cement and also assist in hemostasis is to insert the cement early, while it is viscous. A sponge is then packed into the trough or peg with a hemostat, effectively pressurizing the cement. Removing the sponge will remove a large portion of the cement, but will leave behind cement that is interdigitated within the cancellous bone. This process is repeated three to four times.

Finally, cement is placed only in the trough or pegs with none on the subchondral bone (Fig. 7, B). The glenoid component is then inserted, and thumb pressure is maintained until the cement has hardened. This method allows for excellent pressurization and interdigitation of the cement into the cancellous bone of the glenoid vault (Fig. 7, D). Postoperative radiolucent lines seen with other cementing techniques are eliminated.

HUMERAL IMPLANTATION

Cementing versus press-fit fixation remains controversial. Loosening of the humeral component has been rare regardless of fixation methods.[5,6] Cement use provides for immediate secure fixation in patients with osteoporotic bone. However, in patients with good humeral bone that can safely withstand reaming, a press-fit stem provides secure fixation. This is typically a younger male (younger than 65 years) with osteoarthritis. Regardless of fixation technique, it is essential to insert the prosthesis in the correct version and height. This is determined by trial reductions after the glenoid component is inserted.

Before humeral stem insertion, four drill holes are placed along the rim of the resected humeral head, medial to the lesser tuberosity. Through each drill hole, two #2 braided nonabsorbable sutures are passed and tagged. These are for reattachment of the subscapularis tendon during closure. When cementing the stem, the humeral canal is prepared in typical fashion, using pulse-lavage and drying the canal. Cement is pressurized using a cement delivery system and a canal plug.

SOFT-TISSUE BALANCING

Proper soft-tissue balancing is essential to reestablish the appropriate tension of the deltoid myofascial sleeve. This procedure will maximize mobility as well as stability of the glenohumeral joint.

Subscapularis and Capsular Release With osteoarthritis, the subscapularis and joint capsule become adherent and contracted anteriorly as a result of the progressive loss of external rotation. To regain external rotation postoperatively, the subscapularis needs to be freed as well as lengthened. By taking down the tendon as far laterally as possible during the surgical exposure, maximum tendon length is obtained. During closure, the tendon is repaired back to the humerus in a medial position to its original insertion and secured with #2 nonabsorbable sutures through drill holes (Fig. 5). This step effectively lengthens the tendon. If it does not provide sufficient length, a "Z" lengthening of the tendon should be considered.[7,8]

Before final humeral head size selection, the anterior capsule needs to be resected and the subscapularis muscle released. Using curved Mayo scissors, the medial capsule is separated from the muscle belly and then incised midway between the tendon and the glenoid rim. The capsule is then resected from the glenoid neck and removed. This is performed before glenoid preparation because it allows for better exposure of the glenoid. The capsule is left in place laterally with the tendon to provide stronger tissue for subsequent closure.

The muscle belly of the subscapularis is sharply released down the rotator interval to the base of the coracoid, and then blunt finger dissection is performed, freeing the muscle from the inferior border of the coracoid. Inferiorly, careful separation of the muscle from the inferior capsule will release the subscapularis. Great care must be taken here, because the axillary nerve is in very close proximity to the capsule. The nerve should be identified and protected during this portion of the procedure.

Humeral Head Height Appropriate humeral head size is needed to reestablish the tension of the deltoid myofascial sleeve and avoid instability and weakness. With the head in place there should be approximately 50% head diameter translation anteriorly and posteriorly over the glenoid rim. In addition, the subscapularis tendon must be of sufficient length to be reattached to the humerus and allow for acceptable external rotation with the selected head size. Superiorly, the head size should recreate a smooth transition from the greater tuberosity to the apex of the head to prevent overtensioning of the rotator cuff.

The posterior capsule is often redundant because of posterior subluxation of the arthritic humeral head. If this redundancy creates posterior instability for the glenohumeral joint, then nonabsorbable suture can be used to reef and imbricate the capsule.

CLOSURE

Once there is appropriate soft-tissue tensioning, closure can begin. The subscapularis tendon is securely reattached to the humerus with the #2 nonabsorbable sutures. The rotator interval is closed only at the lateral 1-cm portion to avoid limiting external rotation. The arm is then taken through a range of motion to determine the parameters to be allowed in the postoperative rehabilitation. The deltopectoral interval is closed over drains, followed by skin closure.

The arm is placed in a sling postoperatively. The elbow should be supported on a pillow to avoid extension of the arm, thereby protecting the subscapularis repair.

POSTOPERATIVE REHABILITATION AND MANAGEMENT

A physician-directed therapy program is begun on the first postoperative day. Neer Phase I and II levels of rehabilitation are begun immediately.[9,10] Active motion is allowed in all planes except internal rotation and extension. External rotation is limited to the amount determined intraoperatively that will not jeopardize the subscapularis repair. Supervised passive and active assisted range-of-motion exercises are also initiated on the first postoperative day. Elevation is done in the plane of the scapula, typically without limitation. No resisted exercises or lifting is to be done for 6 weeks while the subscapularis heals. Patients must be cautioned to avoid using their arm to push themselves up in bed or from a chair because this motion requires forceful contraction of the subscapularis.

Patients are instructed on home exercises and precautions. Postoperative range of motion is checked every 2 weeks for the first 6 weeks to monitor progress and start a formal supervised physical therapy program if progress goals are not being met. At 6 weeks, patients can begin internal rotation stretching and gentle resisted exercises. At 12 weeks, all restrictions are lifted, but patients are cautioned not to participate in contact activities or do any aggressive weight training. Annual follow-up visits should be made with serial radiographs to ensure no signs of component failure (Fig. 9).

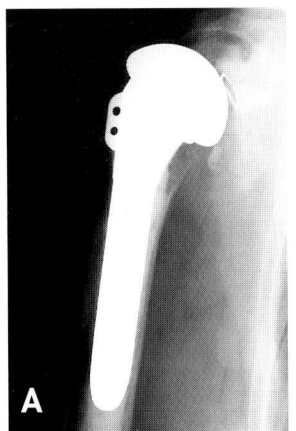

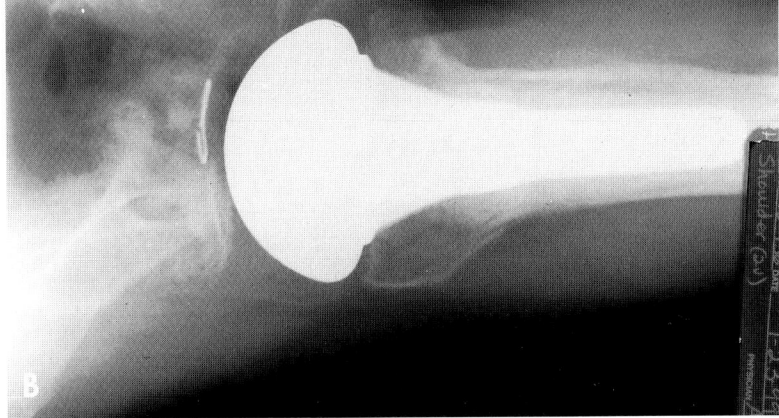

FIGURE 9
Three-month postoperative radiographs of the patient shown in Figure 1. **A,** Anteroposterior radiograph demonstrating a good cement mantle and position of the humeral head relative to the glenoid. **B,** The axillary view demonstrates the humeral head centered within the glenoid. Note there are no radiolucent lines around the glenoid component. Also note there was a nondisplaced greater tuberosity fracture that healed and did not effect the final outcome. The patient was able to actively elevate to 165°, externally rotate to 45°, and internally rotate to the tenth thoracic level. He had no pain.

RESULTS

There have been numerous publications reporting on the success of total shoulder arthroplasty for glenohumeral osteoarthritis.[5-7,9,11-17] Neer[9] reported an 86% excellent or satisfactory result in total shoulder arthroplasty patients. Pain relief was the most predictable outcome. Approximately 90% of patients can be expected to have complete or near complete pain relief.[6,18] Range of motion and function are less predictable and depend on the surgical technique, rotator cuff integrity, and postoperative rehabilitation program.

Torchia and associates[6] analyzed the long-term results of the Neer prosthesis for total shoulder arthroplasties. They determined the probability of prosthesis survival as 93% at 10 years and 87% after 15 years. The patient's age, sex, preoperative diagnosis, condition of the rotator cuff, and preoperative range of motion did not affect the probability of prosthesis survival. The most common cause of failure was glenoid loosening (4%). At an average follow-up of 12.2 years, excellent pain relief was achieved in 83% of patients. Range of motion was significantly improved. Gains were directly related to the condition of the rotator cuff. Humeral loosening was not associated with pain but was seen more frequently with press-fit fixation. At an average radiographic follow-up of 9.6 years, there were no signs of loosening of cement-fixed prostheses; however, the study group was small. In contrast, the press-fit group had a 49% incidence of radiographic loosening. Clinically, there was no pain associated with the loosening. The Neer prosthesis used was a smooth-surfaced design; therefore, it is recommended that if press-fit fixation is going to be used, a tissue-ingrowth type stem be implanted.

The indications for hemiarthroplasty versus total shoulder arthroplasty remain controversial. Concern over loosening of the glenoid component has led some authors to recommend hemiarthroplasty over total shoulder arthroplasty, even in the face of glenoid wear and osteoarthritis.[12,19-21] Sperling and associates,[22,23] however, found that the most common cause of revision surgery for hemiarthroplasty was the development of painful glenoid arthrosis. Levine and associates[24] found that the condition of the glenoid has a significant influence on the success of a hemiarthroplasty. They found that when the glenoid surface is concentric with minimal signs of wear, patients are able to achieve better range of motion than patients with a worn glenoid. Cofield and associates[25] have shown that hemiarthroplasty for glenohumeral osteoarthritis may be effective, but overall is less predictable than total shoulder arthroplasty. In addition, the results may deteriorate over time. Similarly, results from the same institution showed a 97% excellent or satisfactory result for total shoulder arthroplasty[26] as compared to 86% for hemiarthroplasty.[25]

SUMMARY

Total shoulder arthroplasty can provide predictably successful relief of pain and in most instances improve function. Surgical technique, condition of the soft tissues (particularly the rotator cuff), and the postoperative rehabilitation significantly influence successful outcome. Controversies remain, particularly regarding humeral component fixation techniques and indications for glenoid resurfacing. Long-term follow-up studies are necessary to resolve these controversies.

REFERENCES

1. Brems JJ, Yoon HJ, Tetzlaff J: Interscalene block anesthesia and shoulder surgery. *Orthop Trans* 1990;14:250.

2. Brown AR, Weiss R, Greenberg C, Flatow EL, Bigliani LU: Interscalene block for shoulder arthroscopy: Comparison with general anesthesia. *Arthroscopy* 1993;9:295-300.

3. Flatow EL, Bigliani LU: Tips of the trade: Locating and protecting the axillary nerve in shoulder surgery: The tug test. *Orthop Rev* 1992;21:503-505.

4. Flatow EL: Prosthetic design considerations in total shoulder arthroplasty. *Semin Arthroplasty* 1995;6:233-244.

5. Cofield RH: Total shoulder arthroplasty with the Neer prosthesis. *J Bone Joint Surg* 1984;66A: 899–906.

6. Torchia ME, Cofield RH, Settergren CR: Total shoulder arthroplasty with the Neer prosthesis: Long-term results. *J Shoulder Elbow Surg* 1997;6: 495–505.

7. Cofield RH: Degenerative and arthritic problems of the glenohumeral joint, in Rockwood, Matsen (eds): *The Shoulder*. Philadelphia, PA, WB Saunders, 1990, pp 678-749.

8. Bigliani LU, Weinstein DM, Glasgow MT, Pollock RG, Flatow EL: Glenohumeral arthroplasty for arthritis after instability surgery. *J Shoulder Elbow Surg* 1995;4:87–94.

9. Neer CS II, Watson KC, Stanton FJ: Recent experience in total shoulder replacement. *J Bone Joint Surg* 1982;64A:319–337.

10. Hughes M, Neer CS II: Glenohumeral joint replacement and postoperative rehabilitation. *Phys Ther* 1975;55:850–858.

11. Barrett WP, Franklin JL, Jackins SE, Wyss CR, Matsen FA III: Total shoulder arthroplasty. *J Bone Joint Surg* 1987;69A:865–872.

12. Boyd AD Jr, Thomas WH, Scott RD, Sledge CB, Thornhill TS: Total shoulder arthroplasty versus hemiarthroplasty: Indications for glenoid resurfacing. *J Arthroplasty* 1990;5:329–336.

13. Brenner BC, Ferlic DC, Clayton ML, Dennis DA: Survivorship of unconstrained total shoulder arthroplasty. *J Bone Joint Surg* 1989;71A: 1289–1296.

14. Frich LH, Moller BN, Sneppen O: Shoulder arthroplasty with the Neer Mark-II prosthesis. *Arch Orthop Trauma Surg* 1988;107:110–113.

15. Hawkins R, Bell RH, Jallay B: Experience with the Neer total shoulder arthroplasty: A review of 70 cases. *Orthop Trans* 1986;10:232.

16. Hawkins RJ, Bell RH, Jallay B: Total shoulder arthroplasty. *Clin Orthop* 1989;242:188–194.

17. Neer CS II (ed): *Glenohumeral Arthroplasty*. Philadelphia, PA, WB Saunders, 1990, pp 143–271.

18. Schenk T, Iannotti JP: Prosthetic arthroplasty for glenohumeral arthritis with an intact or repairable rotator cuff: Indications, techniques, and results, in Iannotti JP, Williams (eds): *Disorders of the Shoulder: Diagnosis and Management*. Philadelphia, PA, Lippincott Williams & Wilkins, 1999, pp 521–558.

19. Boyd AD Jr, Thornhill TS: Surgical treatment of osteoarthritis of the shoulder. *Rheum Dis Clin North Am* 1988;14:591–611.

20. Brostrom LA, Kronberg M, Wallensten R: Should the glenoid be replaced in shoulder arthroplasty with an unconstrained Dana or St. Georg prosthesis? *Ann Chir Gynaecol* 1992;81:54–57.

21. Clayton ML, Ferlic DC, Jeffers PD: Prosthetic arthroplasties of the shoulder. *Clin Orthop* 1982;164:184–191.

22. Sperling JW, Cofield RH: Revision total shoulder athroplasty for the treatment of glenoid arthrosis. *J Bone Joint Surg* 1998;80:860–867.

23. Sperling JW, Cofield RH, Rowland CM: Neer hemiarthroplasty and Neer total shoulder arthroplasty in patients fifty years old or less: Long-term results. *J Bone Joint Surg* 1998;80:464–473.

24. Levine WN, Djurasovic M, Glasson J, et al: Hemiarthroplasty for glenohumeral osteoarthritis: Results correlated to degree of glenoid wear. *J Shoulder Elbow Surg* 1997;6:449–454.

25. Cofield RH, Frankle MA, Zuckerman JD: Humeral head replacement for glenohumeral arthritis. *Semin Arthroplasty* 1995;6:214–221.

26. Pollock RG, Higgs GB, Codd TP, et al: Total shoulder replacement for the treatment of primary glenohumeral osteoarthritis. *J Shoulder Elbow Surg* 1995;4:S12.

COMPLICATIONS

LYNN A. CROSBY, MD

INTRODUCTION

Complications following total shoulder arthroplasty are rare when compared with those after other major joint replacement surgery. In a recent literature review of 1,183 total shoulder arthroplasties, 123 shoulders (10.4%) were identified as sustaining a complication. It was believed that some of these shoulders had sustained more than one complication; therefore, the overall complication rate for this procedure was somewhat less than 10%.[1]

The most effective means of preventing a complication are meticulous preoperative planning, experience of the surgeon, adherence to sound surgical technique, and intelligent patient selection and education. During the Instructional Course Lecture on shoulder arthroplasty given at the 66th Annual Meeting of the American Academy of Orthopaedic Surgeons it was stated that the average orthopaedic surgeon performs 50 total knee arthroplasties in approximately 3 years. The average orthopaedic surgeon would take 150 years to perform 50 total shoulder arthroplasties.[2] It is difficult for the general orthopaedic surgeon to obtain experience, given these statistics. It is, therefore, essential to make every effort to review surgical planning and patient selection, and when available, to use an orthopaedic surgeon experienced in total shoulder arthroplasty to assist during the surgery to help prevent surgical error and a preventable complication from occurring.

Complications can be subgrouped into those occurring during or after surgery. Postoperative complications are the most frequent and generally are the result of surrounding soft-tissue problems or implant failure. Intraoperative complications are under direct control of the surgeon and can be prevented only by careful and thoughtful surgical practice.

INTRAOPERATIVE COMPLICATIONS

INTRAOPERATIVE FRACTURE

Of the three major intraoperative complications that have been recorded in current reviews of the literature, the most common is intraoperative fracture, which is reported to occur in 0.9% of patients.[3] The fracture most frequently involves the humeral shaft and is the result of torque on the arm producing a spiral fracture of the reamed canal. This complication occurs at one of two critical periods during the surgical procedure. In the reaming process when resistance is met and the assistant has a firm hold of the patient's arm, torque can be generated and a spiral fracture produced. The assistant must be instructed to hold the arm loosely and, if any resistance is felt, to release the grip on the patient's arm allowing the arm to rotate with the hand reamer. The second critical period is during the reduction and dislocation maneuver to test implant stability. Torque again can be produced resulting in a fracture of the humeral shaft. Straight longitudinal distraction must be implemented, and manual assistance to lift the prosthetic humeral head from the joint cavity will prevent the force from being transferred inferiorly into the humeral shaft.

If an intraoperative humeral shaft fracture is sustained, it is essential to stabilize the fracture so it will not interfere with normal postoperative rehabilitation. Generally, the use of a long-stem prosthesis and cerclage wiring will be needed to stabilize the fracture. If the fracture is more distal, the use of standard fracture plate fixation and cerclage wiring may be necessary (Fig. 1). Long-stem prosthesis implants must be part of the preoperative planning if the surgeon is to be prepared to treat this complication effectively.

Fractures of the glenoid are extremely rare and occur most commonly in osteopenic bone, such as that encountered in patients who have rheumatoid arthritis. Most often this complication occurs after the glenoid has been reamed to subchondral bone and the canal prepared to receive a keeled glenoid prosthesis. Retraction on the anterior or posterior glenoid cortex can produce cortical bone failure, and the assistants must be instructed to take care during this critical period. Stable fixation of the fracture is essential to prevent complications of instability of the glenoid component in the postoperative period. Penetration of the glenoid canal may also occur during preparation of the canal with the hand-held burr. Proper orientation is essential to prevent this complication from occurring. Preoperative planning with a good quality axillary radiograph or computed tomography scanning, when needed, is essential to determine if posterior wear of the glenoid is present. Reaming the glenoid to its natural 7° of retroversion and 5° of superior tilt is important to restore the alignment for proper orientation before canal preparation is started. If the cortex is penetrated, bone grafting of the defect is critical and must be performed to prevent cement penetration from occurring. If undetected intraoperatively, this will lead to loosening of the glenoid component (Fig. 2).

NERVE INJURY

Intraoperative injury to the nerve supply to the shoulder girdle is rare (0.6%) but is devastating when it occurs. The axillary nerve is by far the most commonly injured neural structure during shoulder replacement surgery.[4,5] Most of the reported cases in which permanent axillary nerve

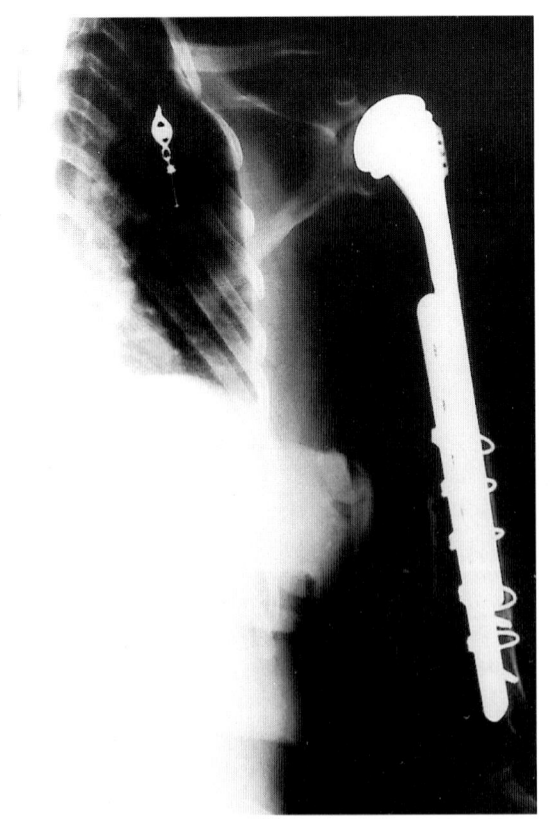

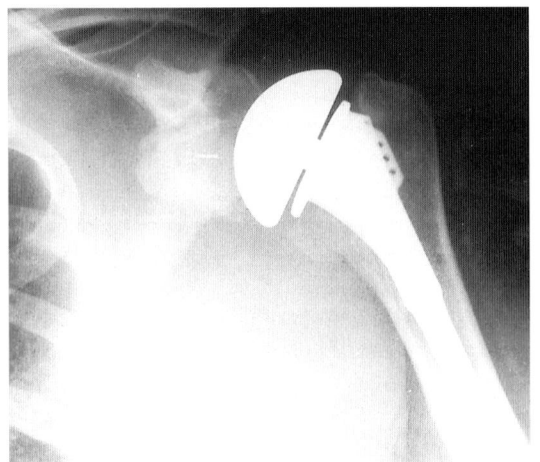

FIGURE 1
Intraoperative fracture treated with long stem implant, plate, cerclage wires, and distal screw fixation.

FIGURE 2
Total shoulder arthroplasty with cement penetration of glenoid cortex which was not addressed at the time of the original surgery. The glenoid component became symptomatically loose and required revision.

injury was diagnosed involved revision surgery or primary surgery on a shoulder that had undergone multiple previous operations. These injuries are secondary to poor tissue plane identification from previous scar formation.[6] Musculocutaneous nerve injury has been reported and usually is related to prolonged retraction on the conjoined tendon complex. Radial nerve injury mostly occurs in conjunction with intraoperative humeral shaft fracture and the subsequent treatment with internal fixation. The radial nerve has been reported to have been injured during extrusion of cement through a defect in the humeral canal. Removal of cement near the nerve has been reported to produce successful recovery.[7] The vast majority of nerve injuries are neurapraxias and will recover with observation. It is critical to complete a neurologic examination of the patient early in the postoperative period and to document any nerve defects. When a nerve injury occurs, a 3- to 6-week period of observation is recommended followed by an electromyographic (EMG) examination if no recovery is noted. The EMG should be repeated at 3 months to differentiate focal from diffuse nerve lesions and to document any recovery. If no recovery has occurred, exploration of the nerve should be considered.[8] There are no large series of cases documenting the results of surgical repair of axillary nerve injuries. Muscle transfer for deltoid dysfunction has not been successful.

MALPOSITIONING OF COMPONENTS

Placing the total shoulder components in less than anatomic position may lead to a decreased range of motion or instability.[9] If the complication is noticed intraoperatively, all attempts to correct the appropriate version should be made. If the components already have been cemented into place, the use of an offset humeral head prosthesis should be considered. This addition to the shoulder arthroplasty options is the most helpful improvement in prosthetic design over the past decade. The offset humeral head allows 5° to 7° of version correction in the anterior or posterior direction (Fig. 3). Before introduction of the offset humeral head component, surgeons were limited

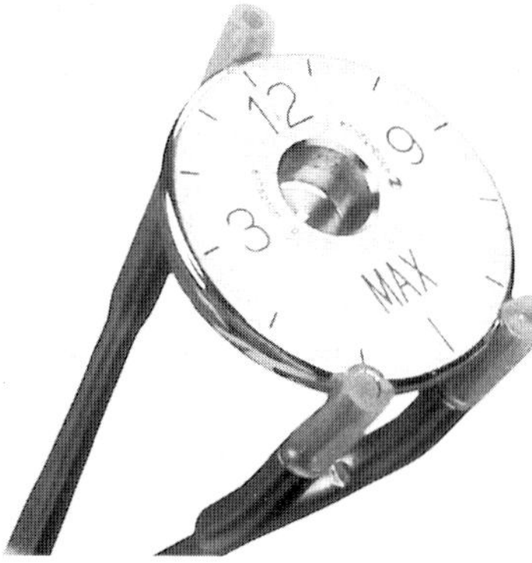

FIGURE 3
Offset humeral head component which allows the surgeon to change the position of the humeral head on the stem component to gain intraoperative stability.

to placing a larger head implant to gain stability or revising the components. The use of large head implants to gain increased stability generally leads to a decreased postoperative range of motion secondary to overstuffing the joint cavity. The long-term complications usually are related to rotator cuff problems secondary to impingement and wearing of the rotator cuff tendon. Immediate revision of malpositioned components usually is the best choice but may lead to a number of complications related to revision surgery.

POSTOPERATIVE COMPLICATIONS

Most complications involving total shoulder arthroplasty occur in the postoperative period. Many of these complications are secondary to surgical error during the initial procedure and can be prevented only by good preoperative planning, sound surgical judgment, and proper patient selection.

INSTABILITY

Component instability may occur in any direction and may be of different degrees of subluxation or dislocation. The exact cause of the instability needs to be carefully evaluated before treatment is recommended. Instability is the second most common complication, occurring in 1.5% of 1,183 shoulder replacement procedures.[1,10]

SUPERIOR MIGRATION

Superior migration of the humeral component is a very common postoperative finding. In one series of 128 total shoulders, superior migration was noted in 23%. Rotator cuff tears were found in only 7 shoulders in this group.[11] There appears to be an imbalance in the force couple between the deltoid and the surgically treated rotator cuff. This imbalance may be due to poor postoperative rehabilitation. If the patient is asymptomatic, he or she should be encouraged to continue to follow the postoperative rehabilitation program. The long-term potential complication of superior migration is loosening of the glenoid component secondary to the "rocking horse mechanism."[12] If the rotator cuff is found to be torn, it should be repaired if possible to prevent this complication.

ANTERIOR INSTABILITY

Anterior instability may be caused by the selection of a smaller than required humeral head component for the amount of joint volume present. The treatment for this intraoperative complication, which was undiagnosed at the time of surgery, is to replace the humeral head with an appropriate sized implant, which also may be an offset type component to gain the needed stability. A torn subscapularis tendon always needs to be considered when evaluating anterior instability following shoulder arthroplasty. The physical examination can be very helpful in determining the status of the subscapularis. If the patient is able to place his or her hand behind her or his back but not able to lift the hand off the body when instructed, the tendon should be considered torn. An alternate physical test is to instruct the patient to place the palm of the hand flat against the abdomen. The examiner attempts to pull the hand away from the abdomen with the patient resisting the pull. If the hand is pulled away easily with very little resistance, the tendon is considered at risk for being torn. Repair of the subscapularis tendon is always required to regain joint stability. If the tendon is not reparable, reconstruction with bone-Achilles tendon allograft as a static restraint has been reported to be successful. If abnormal version of the component is found to be the cause of the increased instability, then revision of the humeral stem should be considered.[10,13,14]

POSTERIOR INSTABILITY

Component malpositioning is the most common cause of posterior instability after shoulder arthroplasty. Failure to recognize and correct posterior wear on the glenoid and, therefore, placing the glenoid component in too much retroversion will cause posterior instability (Fig. 4). Placing the humeral component in too much retroversion will also lead to posterior instability. Revision is advised to correct posterior instability.[10,15] The posterior capsule may be stretched from long standing posterior wear on the glenoid. The capsule may have to be plicated to gain stability after appropriate glenoid reaming has been performed

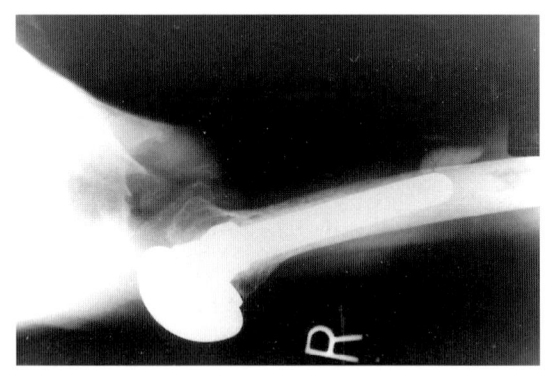

FIGURE 4
Posterior dislocation from malposition of components.

INFERIOR INSTABILITY

Inferior instability is directly related to the loss of normal humeral height. This complication is seen most frequently after treatment of proximal humeral fractures but may occur in elective total shoulder replacement as well. Removing too much of the proximal humerus during resection of the articular surface and not recognizing the loss when the humeral stem is permanently placed will lead to inferior instability. Patients generally have problems elevating the arm past the horizontal plane because of weakness of the deltoid related to shortening of the humerus. Revision surgery is usually necessary to restore the humeral length and regain deltoid strength.[10,14,16]

INFECTION

Infection complicating total shoulder arthroplasty is rare and was found to occur in 5 of 1,183 cases (0.4%)[1] (Fig. 5, A). If the infection is found early in the postoperative period (3 to 6 weeks) and the organism is gram positive, retention of the components is recommended. Early exploration of the wound with judicious irrigation and debridement followed by appropriate parenteral antibiotics has been shown to be an effective treatment. If the organism is gram negative or the infection occurs in the late postoperative period, removal of the implant and all cement is recommended. Placement of antibiotic impregnated beads is used at the time of irrigation and debridment to help sterilize the soft-tissue envelope (Fig. 5, B). The antibiotic should be chosen based on the culture and sensitivity reports. Parenteral antibiotics for 6 weeks followed by implantation of revision components with the use of antibiotics in the cement generally is believed to be an effective treatment.[10]

ROTATOR CUFF TEAR

Tearing of the rotator cuff is the most common complication following total shoulder arthroplasty. The incidence is reported to be 23 of 1,183 or 1.9% of cases. Small tears may be difficult to diagnose, and the patient's complaints of pain may require evaluation with arthrography. Symptomatic tears should be addressed surgically with repair of the rotator cuff in the standard fashion with care to preserve the coracoacromial ligament. Large tears will cause superior subluxation and lead to loosening of the glenoid component from compression forces on the superior rim of the glenoid (Fig. 6). If the tear is asymptomatic the patient should be consulted about the long-term potential complications. Repair of large tears may not be possible. Removing the glenoid component, bone grafting the glenoid cavity defect, and allowing the humeral prosthesis to migrate superiorly has been reported to be an effective form of treat-

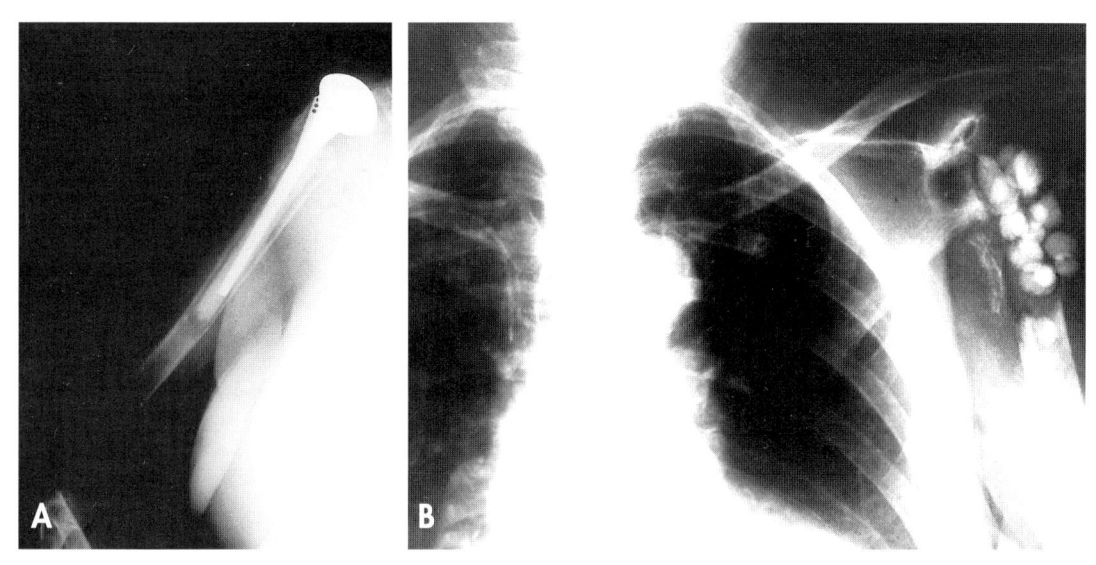

FIGURE 5
A, Lucent lines around cement mantel with bone resorption of the proximal humerus causing loosening of the component secondary to infection. **B,** Removal of an infected total shoulder arthroplasty and placement of antibiotic impregnated beads to help clear a chronic infection.

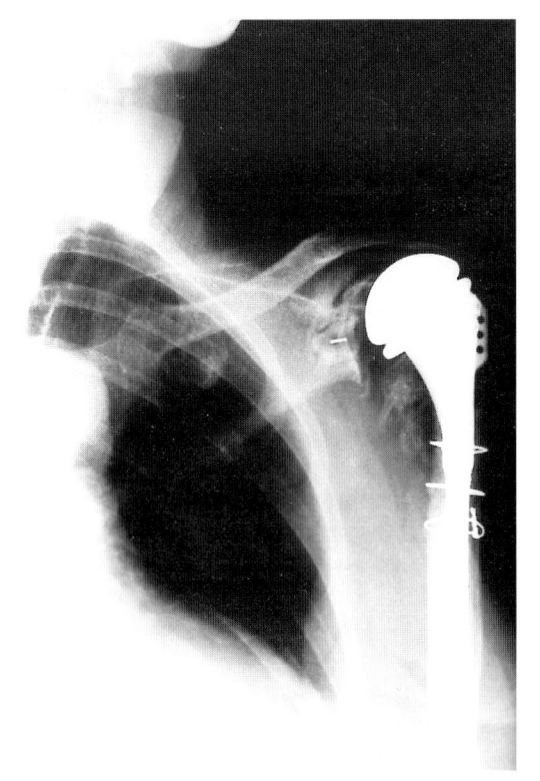

FIGURE 6
Superior migration of the humeral component secondary to large rotator cuff tear with secondary loosening of the glenoid prosthesis. Focus on the superior rim of the stenoid cause the so called "rocking horse" loosening of the component.

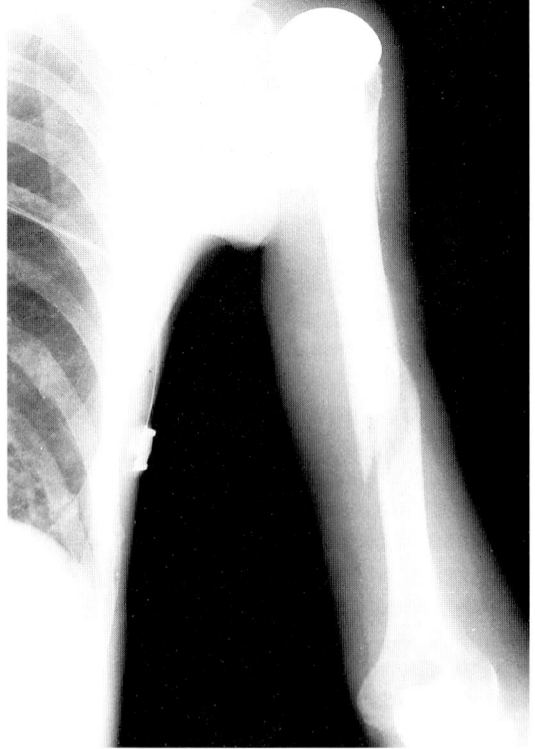

FIGURE 7
Fracture at the tip of the prothesis usually requires revision to a long-stem prosthesis or open reduction and internal fixation if the prosthesis is stable secondary to high nonunion rate with closed treatment.

ment for this difficult clinical situation.[5,9,11] There must be a competent coracoacromial ligament present to give superior stability when performing this salvage procedure.

POSTOPERATIVE FRACTURE

Fractures of the humerus after total shoulder arthroplasty should be considered uncommon but not rare. With the increase in the number of replacement procedures being performed each year, an increase in the number of postoperative fractures should be anticipated. No large series exist to compare closed versus open treatment for this injury. It is widely accepted, however, that if the humeral prosthesis is unstable, a revision to a long-stem prosthesis should be attempted (Fig. 7). Reports of small series of patients suggest improved overall function and a decrease in the nonunion rate with open reduction and internal fixation. Orthoplast fracture bracing also has been shown to produce acceptable results. No current consensus exists because of the small series that presently make up the literature. It is reasonable to suggest a trial of nonsurgical care with fracture bracing unless other factors exist to recommend surgical intervention.[1,5,10]

IMPLANT LOOSENING

When both the humeral and glenoid components are considered together, aseptic loosening is the second most common complication occurring after total shoulder arthroplasty. Glenoid loosening is more common, with 15 cases reported out of 1,183 procedures (1.3%). Radiolucent lines around the bone-cement interface of the glenoid component are very common. These radiolucent lines do not appear to predict a loose component. The progression of the radiolucent lines, however, has correlated with a decrease in function and an increase in pain.

Any shift in position of the glenoid component or circumferential radiolucent lines at least 1.5-mm wide is evidence of a loose glenoid component. Current recommendations to help prevent glenoid loosening center around preserving the subchondral bone plate and using spherical reaming to assure the optimal bone implant interface. The limited use of cement and the avoidance of cement protrusion in the canal and also onto the undersurface of the glenoid component are essential. Humeral prosthesis loosening usually is diagnosed by a change in implant position or a progression of radiolucent lines. Good quality radiographs to compare prosthetic position are essential.[1,5,10]

STIFFNESS

The complication of stiffness rarely is encountered when reviewing large series of total shoulder arthroplasty cases. This situation may represent a lack of reporting of this potentially serious complication. Long-term contracture from years of restricted motion may not be able to be fully returned to normal. It is important for the surgeon to make this clear to the patient preoperatively so there is no misunderstanding on the goals of the procedure. The main reason for replacement surgery of the shoulder remains relief of pain, and no guarantee of a return to normal range of motion should be made to the patient. If stiffness develops in the early postoperative period, the first treatment plan should be an increase in the frequency of physical therapy visits. Manipulation is not a recommended treatment option and can cause tears of the rotator cuff or prosthetic loosening. Open release of contractures is the recommended treatment for progressive loss of motion, with capsulectomy and z-plasty lengthening of the subscapularis if necessary

HETEROTOPIC OSSIFICATION

This not well understood complication is seen rarely in shoulder arthroplasty surgery. It is more common in prosthetic replacement for proximal humeral fractures and especially in head-injured patients. Hetertopic ossification is characterized by the formation of normal bone at ectopic soft-tissue locations.[17] Unless the ossification is extensive, it usually will have little effect on the overall functional result. It does not tend to cause pain, and unless severe restriction of function is encountered the patient can be monitored with serial radiographic evaluation. If surgical intervention is considered for restricted motion, postoperative radiation treatment and the use of indocin have been reported to be beneficial (Fig. 8).

IMPLANT DISSOCIATION

Since the use of modular implants has become popular mainly to help in soft-tissue balancing and revision surgery, complications related to the

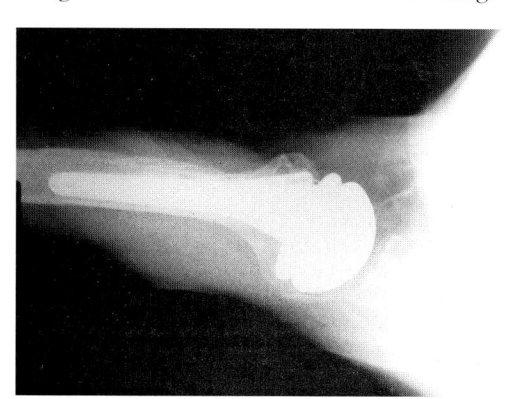

FIGURE 8
Posterior heterotopic ossification after total shoulder arthroplasty.

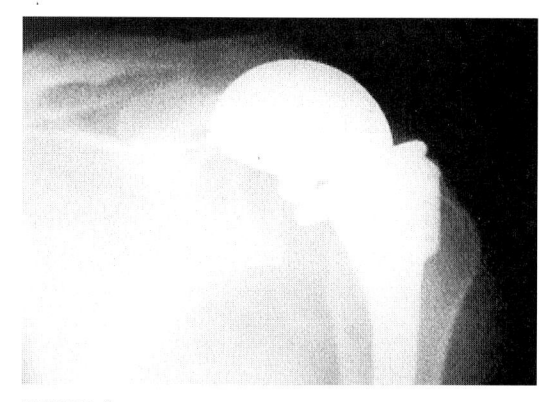

FIGURE 9
Dissociation of the humeral head component from the stem component.

Morse taper components have been reported (Fig. 9). This complication is not related to dislocation of the joint causing dissociation as seen in total hip surgery but rather to moisture between the components not allowing a proper seal to occur between them. It is essential that care is taken to remove all moisture from the Morse taper to prevent this complication. Dissociation may also occur with settling of the humeral stem, which also may interfere with proper seating of the components.[10,18,19]

SUMMARY

This list of complications is a reminder of the potential problems surgeons must deal with in performing surgery intended to improve the quality of the patient's life. If one of these complications occurs, the final result will be compromised, and the patient may be dissatisfied or at least discouraged. It is essential that good communication between the surgeon and patient be established in the preoperative period so the patient is not surprised if a complication does occur.

REFERENCES

1. Cofield RH, Chang W, Sperling JW: Complications of shoulder arthroplasty, in Iannotti JP, Williams GR Jr (eds): *Disorders of the Shoulder: Diagnosis and Management.* Philadelphia, PA, Lippincott Williams & Wilkins, 1999, pp 571–593.
2. Dines DM, Matsen FA, Rockwood CA Jr: Shoulder Arthroplasty: Current Techniques. Proceedings of the American Academy of Orthopaedic Surgeons 66th Annual Meeting, Anaheim, CA. Rosemont, IL, American Academy of Orthopaedic Surgeons, 1999, p 216.
3. Boyd AD Jr, Thornhill T, Barnes CL: Fractures adjacent to humeral prostheses. *J Bone Joint Surg* 1992;74A:1498–1504.
4. Cofield RH: Total joint arthroplasty: The shoulder. *Mayo Clin Proc* 1979;54:500–506.
5. Post M, Grinblat E: Complications of arthroplasty and total joint replacement in the shoulder, in *Complications in Orthopaedic Surgery.*
6. Cofield RH: Unconstrained total shoulder prostheses. *Clin Orthop* 1983;173:97–108.
7. Lynch NM, Cofield RH, Silbert PL, Hermann RC: Neurologic complications after total shoulder arthroplasty. *J Shoulder Elbow Surg* 1996;5:53–61.
8. Miller SR, Bigliani LU: Complications of total shoulder replacement, in Bigliani LU (ed): *Complications of Shoulder Surgery.* Baltimore, MD, Williams & Wilkins, 1993, pp 59–72.
9. Pollock R, Deliz E, McIlveen S, Flatow E, Bigliani L: Prosthetic replacement in rotator cuff deficient shoulders. *J Shoulder Elbow Surg* 1992;1:173–186.
10. Wirth MA, Rockwood CA Jr: Complications of total shoulder-replacement arthroplasty. *J Bone Joint Surg* 1996;78A:603–616.
11. Boyd AD Jr, Aliabadi P, Thornhill TS: Postoperative proximal migration in total shoulder arthroplasty: Incidence and significance. *J Arthroplasty* 1991;6:31–37.
12. Matsen FA III, Arntz CT, Harryman DT II: Rotator cuff tear arthropathy, in Bigliani LU (ed): *Complications of Shoulder Surgery.* Baltimore, MD, Williams & Wilkins, 1993, pp 44–58.
13. Moeckel BH, Altchek DW, Warren RF, Wickiewicz TL, Dines DM: Instability of the shoulder after arthroplasty. *J Bone Joint Surg* 1993;75A;492–497.
14. Wirth MA, Rockwood CA Jr: Glenohumeral instability following shoulder arthroplasty. *Orthop Trans* 1995;19:459.
15. Barrett WP, Franklin JL, Jackins SE, Wyss CR, Matsen FA III: Total shoulder arthroplasty. *J Bone Joint Surg* 1987;69A:865–872.
16. Neer CS II, Watson KC, Stanton FJ: Recent experience in total shoulder replacement. *J Bone Joint Surg* 1982;64A:319–337.
17. Kaplan F, Hahn G, Zasloff M: Heterotopic ossification. *J Am Acad Orthop Surg* 1994;5:288–296.
18. Blevins FT, Deng X, Torzilli PA, Warren RF: Dissociation of modular shoulder arthroplasty components. *Orthop Trans* 1994;18:977.
19. Blevins FT, Deng X, Torzilli PA, Diaes D, Warren R: A biomechanical and implant retrieval study. *J Shoulder Elbow Surg* 1997;2:113–124.

REVISION SHOULDER ARTHROPLASTY

J. MICHAEL WIATER, MD AND WILLIAM N. LEVINE, MD

INTRODUCTION

In 1955, Neer[1] designed a shoulder prosthesis for treatment of proximal humeral defects following fracture-dislocation. By the 1970s, indications for prosthetic replacement of the humeral head were expanded to include primary and secondary osteoarthritis, inflammatory arthritis, osteonecrosis, rotator cuff tear arthropathy, and postcapsulorrhaphy arthropathy. The efficacy of primary shoulder arthroplasty for treatment of a variety of conditions is well established in the literature. Numerous studies have shown a very high percentage of favorable results following primary unconstrained shoulder arthroplasty, with 50% to 100% of patients reporting no or slight pain and demonstrating 29° to 60° improvement in active forward flexion.[2–15]

Approximately 5,000 shoulder arthroplasties per year were performed in the United States from 1990 to 1992.[16] As with other types of arthroplasties, a finite implant life span and complications can lead to revision surgery. Although the rate of revision is low, the number of patients needing revision arthroplasty will continue to increase in the future.

Revision shoulder arthroplasty is an infrequently performed procedure, and little information is available concerning the diagnosis, treatment, and outcome of failed shoulder arthroplasties. The rate of revision of primary shoulder arthroplasties reported in the literature ranges from 5% to 10%.[17] In a review of 22 shoulder arthroplasty series, Matsen and associates[18] found the frequency of reoperation to be 7%. In 1982, Neer and Kirby[19] published the first series addressing failed shoulder arthroplasties requiring revision. They found that the causes of failure were multiple in this series of 40 patients, which included both failed constrained and failed unconstrained arthroplasties. Most were treated with conversion to unconstrained total shoulder arthroplasties. Satisfactory pain relief and function for the activities of daily living were obtained in all but five patients. Cofield and Edgerton[17] reviewed the complications of total shoulder arthroplasty and their experience with 79 revision arthroplasties, but believed that a detailed analysis of results was not possible because of the many different reasons for failure and the variety of treatment methods used.

Some authors have included limited discussions of the small numbers of revisions in their published series of shoulder arthroplasties.[2,8,9,14,15,20] In a prospective series of 50 total shoulder arthroplasties, Barrett and associates[5] revised four arthroplasties (8%). Three of the four had minimum pain at latest follow-up. Torchia and associates[15] revised 11 of 113 prostheses (10%), but did not separately report the results of these patients. Arntz and associates[3] revised the components of three out of 19 patients with irreparable tears of the rotator cuff who developed marked pain after the primary arthroplasty. At latest follow-up, all three patients had pain only after unusual activities and had maintained their prerevision range of motion.

The outcome after revision of unconstrained shoulder arthroplasties is generally inferior to the outcome to be expected after primary arthroplasty. Revision surgery is technically demanding, and the causes of prosthesis failure are often multifactorial and difficult to diagnose accurately before surgery. A shoulder arthroplasty may require revision because of problems with the soft tissues, the bony structures, the implant itself, or a combination of these. The multiple factors responsible for prosthesis failure and the various types of revision operations that may be performed make it difficult to draw universal conclusions regarding failed shoulder arthroplasty. Because it is so infrequently performed, few centers have had extensive experience with revision shoulder arthroplasty. Consequently, little information exists in the literature with which to formulate treatment guidelines. Reported complications of primary shoulder arthroplasty that may lead to revision surgery are myriad and include component loosening, instability, rotator cuff tearing, periprosthetic fracture, deltoid dysfunction, infection, failure of the implant, soft-tissue adhesions and scarring, and tuberosity malunion or nonunion.

PREOPERATIVE EVALUATION

The preoperative evaluation of the patient with a painful shoulder arthroplasty must first determine the cause of the pain. Second, whether or not a surgical solution to the problem exists must be determined. Finally, it must be decided whether or not the patient is a candidate for revision surgery.

HISTORY

The preoperative evaluation begins with a complete history. Important information to collect includes the initial diagnosis that ultimately led to arthroplasty, a complete surgical history of the shoulder both before and after the failed arthroplasty, the type of prosthesis implanted, and the details of the postoperative rehabilitation program.[21] The timing of the onset of pain in relation to the primary arthroplasty is important. No improvement in symptoms immediately following arthroplasty may be suggestive of acute infection, instability, or inadequate soft-tissue releases. A period of satisfactory function after primary arthroplasty followed by deterioration could be consistent with delayed infection, aseptic loosening, or glenoid arthrosis. The treating surgeon should try to obtain any prior radiographs, old surgical reports, or office notes. Knowledge of the previous method of surgical management is helpful in planning the surgical reconstruction. As with any failed joint arthroplasty, the clinician should have a high index of suspicion for infection, and the patient should be questioned about any history of fever, chills, wound healing problems after surgery, or recent invasive procedures.

PHYSICAL EXAMINATION

The physical examination begins with an inspection of the shoulder at rest. Muscular atrophy or defects are assessed as is the overall attitude and posture of the shoulder. The deltoid muscle should be examined closely for evidence of denervation or detachment. Scars from the previous surgery are noted. A prominent humeral prosthesis may indicate anterosuperior instability. Next, the range of passive and active motion in elevation, abduction, external rotation, and internal rotation is measured. Hawkins and associates[22] found that a "clunk" during forward elevation is suggestive of a loose glenoid component. It should be determined, if possible, whether limited motion results from contracture of the soft tissues or from mechanical impingement of the implant and bone. Strength measurements provide information about the integrity of the rotator cuff. The degree and direction of instability are assessed. Finally, a detailed neurologic examination is performed. Function of the brachial plexus and all peripheral nerves is tested, with particular attention paid to the axillary, musculocutaneous, radial, and suprascapular nerves. Any nerve deficits should be further evaluated with a complete electrodiagnostic study.

DIAGNOSTIC STUDIES

Standard radiographs for all patients include anteroposterior views perpendicular to the plane of the scapula taken in neutral, internal, and external rotation; a lateral scapular 'Y' view; and an axillary view. A high quality set of standard radiographs is sufficient for preoperative planning in the great majority of cases of failed shoulder arthroplasty, making additional studies unnecessary. In all cases, serial radiographs should be examined to follow the progression of radiolucent lines, osteolysis, implant position, and stability. Spot radiographs with fluoroscopic guidance may be useful for demonstrating radiolucencies at the cement-bone interface.[23]

Computed tomography (CT) scans may be obtained on an individual basis, because the quality of the study is lessened by metallic artifact. However, newer digital subtraction techniques may be used to allow assessment of bone.[24,25] CT can delineate the bony anatomy in detail, particularly the status of the articular surfaces and the relationships between the tuberosities, shaft, head, and glenoid. It is especially helpful for assessing posterior glenoid wear when the axillary radiograph is inconclusive. Three-dimensional reconstructions may be helpful in select complex cases. Arthrography is useful for demonstrating prosthetic loosening or tearing of the rotator cuff.

Infection should be ruled out before recommending revision surgery, particularly in those who have had continuous pain since a previous arthroplasty. A sedimentation rate and white blood cell count with differential are good laboratory screening measures. A C-reactive protein level is useful if acute infection is suspected. If the history and laboratory studies suggest the possibility of infection, the joint should be aspirated and fluid sent for culture. Indium-labeled white blood cell scans may be helpful if other studies are inconclusive and clinical suspicion remains high. If suspicious fluid or tissue is encountered at the time of arthroplasty, more cultures should be taken and tissue sent to pathology for frozen sections. The presence of many white blood cells per high power field on frozen section analysis is strong evidence for underlying infection.[26] If this happens, the revision arthroplasty should be discontinued and the infection treated.

Shoulder arthroscopy has been described to diagnose glenoid component loosening when plain radiographs are inconclusive.[27] While viewing with the arthroscope through the standard posterior portal, a probe can be placed through an anterior portal to lever against the glenoid component. Movement of the component confirms loosening.

SPECIFIC INDICATIONS

The main indication for revision shoulder arthroplasty is pain relief. Restoration of motion, strength, function, and stability are secondary indications, because achievement of these goals is somewhat less predictable. Patients with failed shoulder arthroplasty and mild disability are best managed with conservative treatment. Likewise, elderly and sedentary patients or those with limited functional demands may not be good surgical candidates. Physical therapy emphasizing range of motion and strengthening of the rotator cuff, deltoid, and scapular stabilizers should be initiated. Nonsteroidal anti-inflammatory medications may offer some pain relief. Motivated patients with more severe disability and pain who have failed conservative measures may benefit from revision arthroplasty. Before surgery, however, the surgeon must have a discussion with the patient emphasizing that results after repeat arthroplasty are rarely as good as results after primary arthroplasty. The importance of compliance with the postoperative rehabilitation program should be stressed. Failure to attend therapy sessions or noncompliance with the rehabilitation protocol can jeopardize any gains achieved at the time of surgery.

LOOSENING

Loosening of the glenoid component is the most common cause of failure leading to revision of total shoulder arthroplasty.[28] Symptomatic loosening of a glenoid component is treated by removal of the component. In rare circumstances, a new component may be cemented in place if adequate glenoid bone stock is available in the face of a functional deltoid and rotator cuff. In most cases, these conditions are not met and the glenoid component is removed. Large glenoid defects may be bone grafted primarily to provide a stable base for the glenohumeral fulcrum. If a well-fixed modular humeral component has been used and the prosthesis height and version are appropriate, the modular head may be removed to allow access to the glenoid.[29] In this situation, the original implant system instrumentation must be available with a variety of modular humeral head sizes to allow for soft-tissue balancing, because the original head size may be too small once the glenoid component is removed. If a one-piece humeral component has been used, it will likely need to be removed to obtain adequate glenoid exposure. Once exposed, loose glenoid components can be removed easily with a rongeur. Solidly fixed polyethylene glenoid components can be removed by separating the glenoid face from the keel with a sharp osteotome.[24] The keel is then removed from the vault with flexible osteotomes or a high-speed burr. O'Driscoll and associates[0] have recently reported good results in a small series of patients treated with arthroscopic removal of loosened polyethylene glenoid components. While viewing through the posterior portal, a sharp narrow osteotome is used to cut the glenoid into pieces, which are then extracted through the anterior portal.

While rare, loosening of the humeral component does occur (Fig. 1). As previously men-

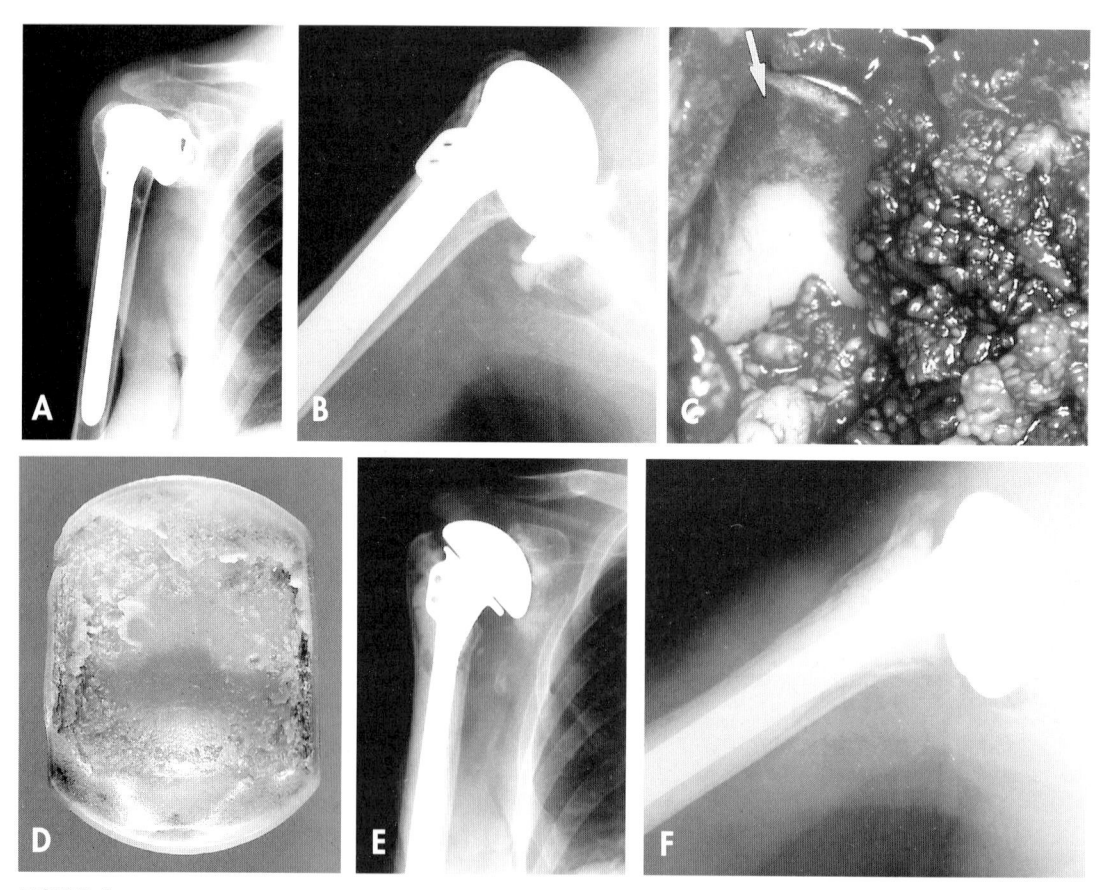

FIGURE 1

A, Severe humeral osteolysis and subsidence of an uncemented humeral component is present 15 years after total shoulder arthroplasty in this 56-year-old woman with rheumatoid arthritis. **B,** Axillary radiograph demonstrates probable glenoid component loosening. **C,** At revision arthroplasty, polyethylene wear (arrow), metallosis, and hypertrophic synovitis were present. Both components were grossly loose. **D,** Retrieved glenoid component shows heavy wear and delamination. **E** and **F,** Postoperative radiographic appearance after glenoid component removal and revision to a cemented long-stem humeral prosthesis.

tioned, recent evidence has suggested that uncemented humeral prostheses may have a higher rate of loosening at intermediate-term follow-up than prostheses implanted with modern cementing techniques.[15,31-33] Because of this and the fact that humeral bone stock is often less than optimal when revision of the humeral component is necessary, we believe that revision to an uncemented humeral prosthesis is rarely indicated in cases of aseptic loosening.

GLENOID ARTHROSIS AFTER HUMERAL HEMIARTHROPLASTY

Painful glenoid arthrosis is the most common indication for revision arthroplasty following humeral head replacement[28,31] (Fig. 2). Exposure of the glenoid may be difficult because of obstruction by the humeral component and soft-tissue scarring. Once a glenoid component is implanted, a smaller humeral head size often is needed to accommodate the thickness of the polyethylene and prevent overstuffing the joint.

With the humeral head in place, 50% anterior and posterior translation on the face of the glenoid should be possible.[26]

INFECTION

Diagnosis of shoulder prosthetic infection may be difficult. Diagnostic and laboratory studies may be inconclusive, and patients may exhibit few constitutional symptoms.[28,34] Eradication of delayed deep prosthetic infection requires removal of the prosthesis and all of the methylmethacrylate cement mantle. At surgery, prophylactic antibiotic administration should be withheld until deep cultures are taken. Extended humeral osteotomy may be necessary to remove the prosthesis and/or distal cement. If a low-virulence organism is responsible, a one-stage resection arthroplasty and debridement followed by immediate reimplantation with antibiotic impregnated cement may be considered.[34] In most cases, a high-virulence organism is responsible, and two-stage reconstruction is advised.

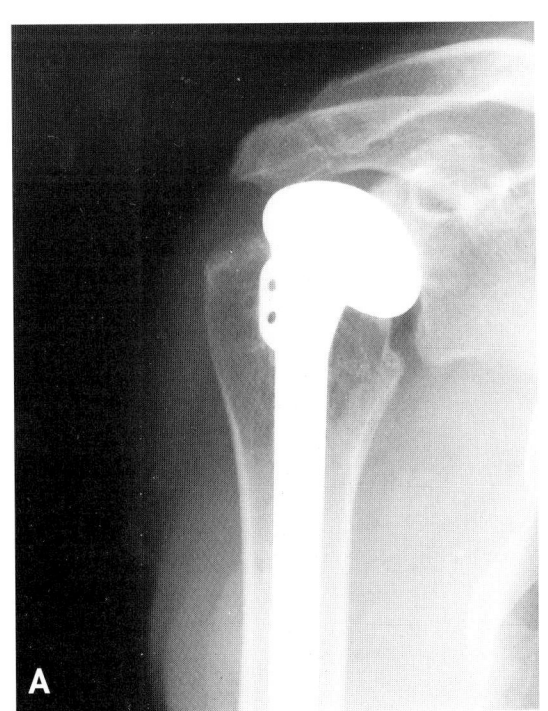

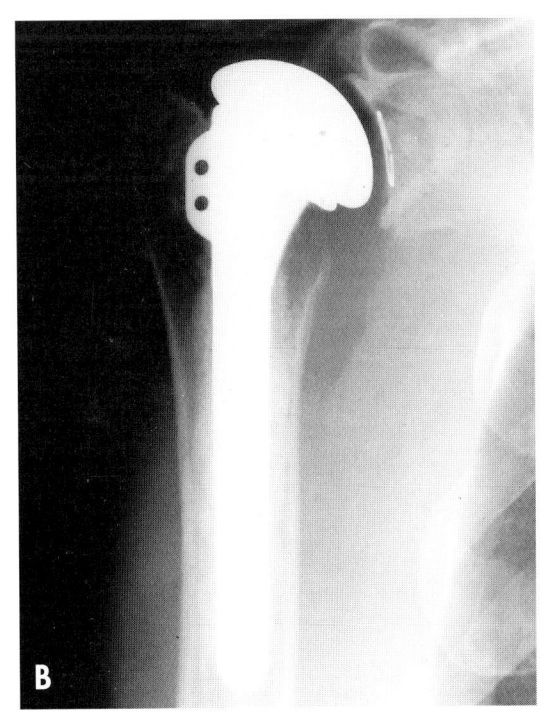

FIGURE 2
A, Painful glenoid arthrosis developed in this 65-year-old man 4 years after uncemented humeral hemiarthroplasty. **B,** Revision to a cemented modular total shoulder arthroplasty resulted in significant pain relief.

We typically treat the patient with home intravenous antibiotics tailored to the sensitivity of the organism for 4 to 6 weeks. Antibiotic impregnated cement spacers may be used to provide local antibiotic delivery and maintain soft-tissue sleeve length.[35,36] Studies have shown Palacos (Zimmer, Warsaw, IN) cement to have superior antibiotic elution properties.[37] Reimplantation is delayed for a minimum of 6 to 8 weeks, provided the white blood cell count, erythrocyte sedimentation rate, and C-reactive protein have returned to acceptable levels.

FAILED HUMERAL HEMIARTHROPLASTY FOR FRACTURE

Multiple factors may lead to failure of a humeral hemiarthroplasty for severe proximal humeral fracture. Tuberosity malunion may cause painful subacromial impingement. If superior displacement of the tuberosity is mild, anterior acromioplasty may provide adequate decompression of the subacromial space. Severe displacement may necessitate tuberosity osteotomy and repair, although this is a less desirable option because healing of tuberosity to its new position is not guaranteed. Tuberosity nonunion can lead to loss of motion and weakness and even superior humeral migration from compromise of the rotator cuff. Surgical intervention usually is warranted in symptomatic cases. Again, achieving bony union between the tuberosity and the shaft is difficult. Rigid fixation is mandatory, and consideration should be given to supplemental bone grafting.

Determination of the proper humeral head height is difficult in the fracture setting because of bony destruction and loss of the normal anatomic landmarks (Fig. 3). Positioning the head too proximally places the rotator cuff tendons under excessive stress. This stress may lead to attritional wear of the tendon against the prominent prosthetic head. Eventually, the rotator cuff tendon may rupture. If this occurs, repair of the rotator cuff without addressing the component malposition is doomed to failure. The humeral prosthesis must be revised to a more acceptable height in addition to repair of the rotator cuff. Conversely, excessively low head height leads to loss of humeral length. Inferior subluxation and limitation of overhead motion result from functional lengthening of the deltoid muscle and loss of power.[19]

INSTABILITY

Glenohumeral instability following arthroplasty can occur in the anterior, posterior, superior, and

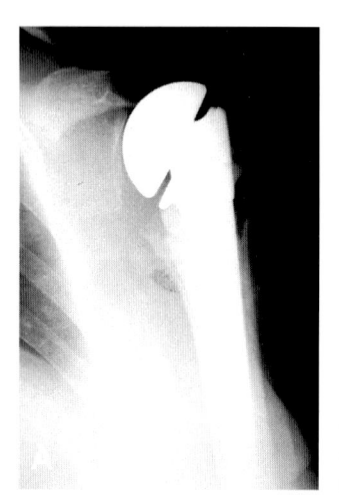

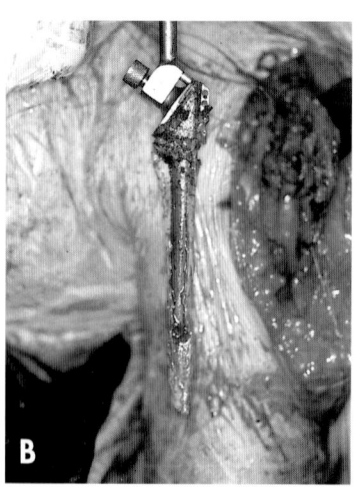

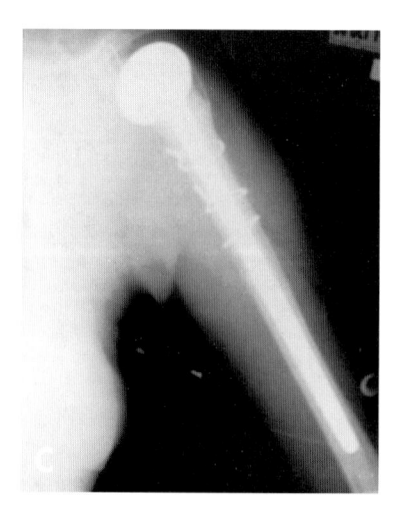

FIGURE 3
A, Excessive humeral head height 2 years after hemiarthroplasty for four-part proximal humeral fracture led to limited motion and painful subacromial impingement in this 58-year-old woman. **B,** Extraction of the well-fixed cemented humeral component was difficult and required extended humeral osteotomy. **C,** At surgery, most of the glenoid was devoid of cartilage. Revision to a cemented long-stem total shoulder arthroplasty was performed.

inferior directions, or in a combination thereof. It may occur to any degree, from mild subluxation to severe dislocation. The chronicity of the instability is important. Early instability may be caused by malposition of the components or rupture of the subscapularis repair. Multiple causes may be responsible, including rotator cuff tearing, severe soft-tissue contracture on the side of the joint opposite the instability, disruption of the coracoacromial arch, failed subscapularis repair, component loosening causing a shift in position, oversized or undersized components, and component malposition. Revision of a subluxated or dislocated shoulder arthroplasty often requires correction of prosthetic malposition, bone grafting, and soft-tissue balancing. Failure to address all contributing factors will lead to recurrence of the instability. In some cases, instability resulting from small amounts of abnormal version in well-fixed modular humeral components can be overcome by upgrading the size of the humeral head, avoiding the potential destruction of the proximal humerus that could occur with revision of the humeral stem.

Anterior instability can result from excessive anteversion of the humeral component, anterior deltoid dysfunction, or rupture of the subscapularis repair.[38,39] Of these, rupture of the subscapularis repair is the most common. Failure of the subscapularis repair may result from attritional wear on the undersurface of the tendon by an oversized humeral head component, poor tissue quality, aggressive rehabilitation, or inadequate repair. Moeckel and associates[39] reviewed 236 shoulder arthroplasties, of which 10 had postoperative instability. Seven of the shoulders were unstable anteriorly because of dehiscence of the subscapularis. Four were treated with primary repair. The remaining three, however, required anterior static restraint reconstruction with Achilles tendon allograft.

Anterosuperior instability is the direct result of an incompetent coracoacromial arch.[40] Previous surgery, excessive acromioplasty, or coracoacromial ligament resection may compromise the buffering effect of the coracoacromial arch and allow the humeral prosthesis to migrate superiorly by the upward pull of the deltoid muscle, especially in the setting of a weak or nonfunctional rotator cuff. Premature loosening of the glenoid component, if present, is likely to occur because of edge loading at the superior glenoid rim.[5] Anterosuperior instability after arthroplasty presents a difficult surgical dilemma, because results of coracoacromial arch reconstructive procedures have been uniformly poor.[40,41] This type of instability is to be differentiated from superior humeral migration that may result from a deficient rotator cuff, a proud humeral prosthesis, or, rarely, an inferiorly placed glenoid component. In this situation, the humeral head rides high but is confined by an intact coracoacromial arch. Surgical options for superior humeral migration have more predictable results and include rotator cuff repair and humeral component revision. Repair of the rotator cuff coupled with superior transposition of the subscapularis tendon above the equator of the humeral head centers the humeral head within the glenoid by restoring the head-depressing effect of the rotator cuff. Active elevation is improved as the glenohumeral fulcrum is reestablished, even if complete coverage of the humeral head is not possible.

Posterior instability is associated with a tight anterior soft-tissue repair, uncorrected posterior glenoid erosion, retroversion of the glenoid component beyond 20°, or retroversion of the humeral component more than 45°.[10,16] Excessive posterior glenoid erosion is seen in the setting of chronic locked posterior dislocation, longstanding severe osteoarthritis, and after prior repair of anterior instability. It is best recognized on axillary radiographs. Anatomic glenoid version may be restored by careful lowering of the anterior glenoid during reaming. Severe deficiencies may require glenoid bone grafting techniques.[42] If instability is a result of malversion of the prosthesis, the component is revised to the appropriate version and cemented in place. Chronic posterior instability leads to lax and redundant posterior capsule. The excess posterior joint volume should be reduced by capsular plication.

Inferior instability in the immediate postoperative period after shoulder replacement is usually due to deltoid atony and often resolves spontaneously with time and rehabilitation. However, inferior subluxation after humeral head replacement for proximal humeral fracture may be the result of inadequate restoration of humeral length. Loss of bony landmarks and severe soft-tissue damage make determination of appropriate humeral length extremely difficult. Active elevation is severely affected as the deltoid and rotator cuff muscles are functionally lengthened and thus weakened. During fracture cases, humeral length can be restored by tensioning the myofascial sleeve with longitudinal traction during trialing (placing a trial component to determine the fit and then replacing it with the permanent implant) of the humeral component. The surgeon should aim to place the prosthetic head slightly higher than the tuberosities.

PERIPROSTHETIC FRACTURE

Satisfactory results have been reported following both surgical and nonsurgical management of periprosthetic humeral fractures.[43–47] However, the trend is toward early surgical intervention in most instances. Based on analysis of nine humeral fractures occurring in a series of 499 shoulder arthroplasties, Wright and Cofield[47] classified periprosthetic humeral shaft fractures into three types. Type A fractures extend proximally from the tip of the prosthesis, type B fractures are centered at the tip of the prosthesis, and type C fractures involve the humeral shaft distal to the prosthesis. Surgical options include cerclage wiring, cemented long-stem prosthesis with cerclage wiring, or open reduction and internal fixation with plate, screws, and cerclage wiring. Autogenous bone grafting is recommended.

Intraoperative fractures should be repaired at the time of arthroplasty with cerclage wiring and a long-stem prosthesis extending at least two cortical diameters beyond the fracture. Treatment of postoperative fractures depends on the fracture type. Type A fractures may disrupt a significant portion of the bone-implant interface and lead to implant loosening. In this situation, revision arthroplasty and stabilization of the fracture is indicated. Type B fractures may be treated with a fracture orthosis if acceptable alignment can be achieved. If good alignment is not possible or if delayed union occurs, open reduction and internal fixation without prosthesis revision is advised, using a plate, screws, and cerclage wiring. Type C fractures usually heal with immobilization and should be managed according to guidelines for distal humeral fractures.

SURGICAL TECHNIQUE

Revision shoulder arthroplasty is considered one of the most difficult shoulder reconstructive procedures.[19,48] Bone loss and soft-tissue scarring, contracture, and deficiency create a technical challenge. Meticulous surgical technique and adherence to surgical principles specific to shoulder reconstruction are mandatory, including careful dissection and mobilization of the soft tissues, release of contracted rotator cuff tendons, preservation of the posterior rotator cuff attachment and of the coracoacromial arch, and proper implant positioning.

Revision shoulder arthroplasty is performed with the patient in the beach chair position. An extended deltopectoral skin incision is used, using the previous skin incision if possible. If use of the previous skin incision would make a deltopectoral approach difficult, a new skin incision should be made. It has been our experience that skin flap necrosis at the intersection of new skin incisions with old surgical scars is extremely rare when operating about the shoulder because of the excellent vascularity of the soft tissues. The deltopectoral interval is developed, and generous skin flaps are undermined. If the interval is scarred and difficult to locate, dissection should begin proximally or distally, where the tissue planes are uninvolved, and proceed toward the center of the incision. We routinely take the cephalic vein laterally with the deltoid muscle. Adhesions in the subacromial and subdeltoid space are released bluntly. The coracohumeral ligament is often contracted, limiting external rotation, and should be released at the base of the coracoid. At this point, the axillary nerve should be identified and palpated at the inferior border of the subscapularis. The "tug test"[49] is useful when scarring and altered anatomy make identification of the nerve difficult. Once the axillary nerve is identified, it must be protected and periodically reexamined throughout the procedure. Following release from the lesser tuberosity, the subscapularis is tagged with heavy sutures. The inferior capsule is released from the humeral neck as the arm is externally rotated and the humeral component is gently dislocated. Bone quality is often poor in the revision setting, and the dislocation maneuver should never be forceful for fear of fracturing the humerus. Difficulty dislocating the humerus is usually due to inadequate soft-tissue releases. In rare cases only, detachment of the anterior deltoid from the clavicle and anterior acromion may be necessary.

Removal of well-fixed cemented or porous-ingrowth humeral prostheses may require the use of shoulder prosthesis extraction equipment specific to the manufacturer, ultrasonic cement removal devices, hip revision arthroplasty instruments, and high-speed drills. If these devices fail, we have found extended humeral osteotomy to be an effective and efficient means of removing a solidly fixed humeral component without destroying the humerus (Fig. 4). The anterior humerus is exposed subperiosteally with needle-point electrocautery proximally in the interval between the deltoid tendon laterally and the pectoralis tendon medially, and distally in the interval between the triceps muscle laterally and the brachialis muscle medially. Using a microsagittal saw, longitudinal cuts are made so as to remove a section of the anterior humerus. This cortical section should measure roughly one third of the circumference of the humerus. A final transverse cut is made distally. The osteotomy should extend distally to within 3 to 4 cm of the tip of the distal cement plug to allow ease of extraction of the prosthesis and cement. After the cuts are made, the cortical section of bone is gently pried loose with wide thin osteotomes, taking care to avoid fracturing it. The prosthesis then usually can be removed with a slaphammer or mallet without much difficulty. At this point, the humerus should be manipulated with great caution to avoid fracturing through the osteotomy. After the distal medullary cement and any cement on the osteotomized cortical section are removed, the humerus is prepared for reimplantation. The osteotomized section is replaced and secured with at least three cerclage wires. We prefer to cement a long-stem humeral prosthesis in the revision setting. The tip of the prosthesis should extend at least two cortical diameters beyond the osteotomy, which is a significant stress riser.

Proper management of the soft-tissue problems present when treating a failed shoulder arthroplasty is of paramount importance. Limited motion is nearly universal, resulting from a combination of contracture and scarring of the deltoid, rotator cuff, and capsule. If the deltoid origin is detached and retracted, it should be carefully mobilized to avoid injury to the axillary nerve and should be securely reattached to the acromion. If the subscapularis is contracted and limits external rotation, as is frequently the case, several techniques exist to restore length. If external rotation is limited to 30° or less, the subscapularis should be taken directly off the bone as laterally as possible to gain length. A complete 360° release of the subscapularis tendon is performed by sharply releasing adherent anterior capsule from the undersurface of the tendon with scissors once a plane is developed bluntly between the capsule and the subscapularis. Any adhesions to the base of the coracoid process or overlying coracoid strap muscles are released as well. The release is judged complete when the subscapularis tendon has an elastic or springy feel when the surgeon pulls on the traction sutures, as would be expected from a functional musculotendinous unit. The insertion of the subscapularis is medialized by repairing it to the osteomized humeral neck with heavy transosseous sutures, allowing further gain in functional length. If external rotation is limited to neutral or less, a coronal-plasty lengthening may be necessary, provided the tendon and capsule are of sufficient quality.[35] As a rule of thumb, every centimeter gain in length of the anterior tissues increases external rotation by 20°. If internal rotation is restricted, the posterior capsule should be released just lat-

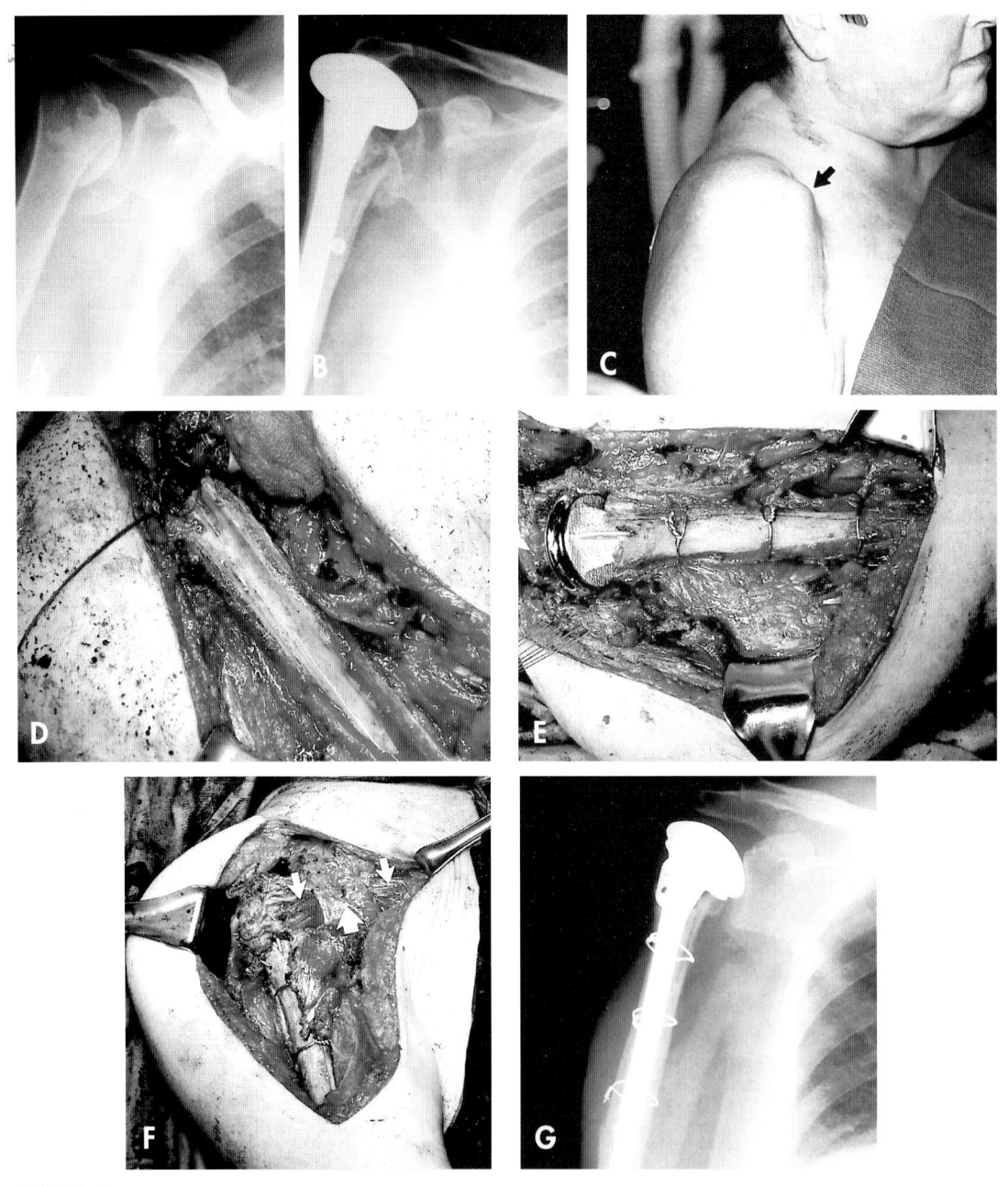

FIGURE 4

A, This 46-year-old woman sustained a head-splitting proximal humeral fracture and was treated with a humeral hemiarthroplasty. An excessively proud prosthesis lead to a massive rotator cuff tear. Reoperation was performed, consisting of rotator cuff repair, acromioplasty, and coracoacromial ligament resection. **B,** Radiographic appearance at the time of referral to our institution. Prosthetic malposition and anterosuperior instability are evident. **C,** On physical examination, the prosthetic humeral head (arrow) was palpable beneath the skin. **D,** Revision shoulder arthroplasty was performed. Appearance after extended humeral osteotomy and removal of the humeral component. **E,** The osteotomy was repaired with cerclage wires and a longstem prosthesis was cemented. **F,** To prevent anterosuperior instability and substitute for a deficient rotator cuff, the pectoralis major (arrows pointing down) was transferred to the proximal humerus underneath the coracoid strap muscles (arrow pointing up). **G,** Postoperative radiographic appearance at 4 months follow-up. Note maintenance of acromiohumeral interval.

eral to the glenoid attachment. Release of the inferior capsule from the humeral neck restores abduction.

Small tears of the rotator cuff tendon should be repaired to bone with transosseous sutures. Larger tears of the rotator cuff should be mobilized and repaired if possible. Intra- and extracapsular releases may be necessary to gain lateral excursion of the rotator cuff tendon. The coracoacromial arch provides the only restraint to superior humeral migration in the severely rotator cuff-deficient shoulder.[40] If a large to massive rotator cuff tear is present, the coracoacromial arch should not be violated or anterosuperior instability may result. At this time, anterosuperior instability has no viable surgical solution.[41]

OTHER SURGICAL OPTIONS

The success of shoulder arthroplasty has markedly diminished the indications for glenohumeral fusion and resection arthroplasty. However, these salvage procedures continue to play a role in the management of the patient with a failed shoulder arthroplasty and should be included in the discussion with any patient considering revision shoulder arthroplasty.

GLENOHUMERAL FUSION

Glenohumeral fusion is rarely indicated for the treatment of primary arthritic conditions of the shoulder. For the patient with a failed shoulder arthroplasty, fusion may be offered in cases of severe bone loss, chronic low-grade infection, failed multiple revision arthroplasties, intractable instability, or extensive deficiency of the rotator cuff, deltoid, or coracoacromial arch.[19,50]

Results of shoulder fusion have been variable. Patients are often dissatisfied with the results of fusion and complain of limited function. Interestingly, pain is not always relieved. Hawkins and Neer[51] found that half the patients in their series of 17 successful fusions still complained of pain, none could use the extremity overhead, and most had difficulties with hygiene.[51] However, other investigators have reported satisfactory rates as high as 80% after shoulder fusion.[52,53]

RESECTION ARTHROPLASTY

Resection arthroplasty may be considered for failed arthroplasty patients with resistant prosthetic infection, intractable pain, or extensive bone or soft-tissue loss in which reimplantation is contraindicated.[19] Although pain may be relieved in some cases, range of motion and function are uniformly poor as the fulcrum of the shoulder is lost.[54,55] Active forward elevation is typically limited to 40° to 90°, and internal and external rotation is markedly diminished.[55] Like glenohumeral fusion, resection arthroplasty has no role today in the treatment of primary arthritic conditions of the shoulder.

REVIEW OF THE LITERATURE

Peer-reviewed literature specifically dealing with revision shoulder arthroplasty is sparse. The first report by Neer and Kirby[19] in 1982 prospectively reviewed 40 consecutive revision arthroplasties in 36 patients. Three revisions of failed constrained arthroplasties were done; the remainder were revisions of failed unconstrained arthroplasties. Revision procedures performed included Neer II unconstrained arthroplasty in 34 shoulders, arthrodesis in three, resection arthroplasty in two, and Neer fixed-fulcrum arthroplasty in one shoulder. Results were reported only for the shoulders revised to an unconstrained arthroplasty. Of these, all but five (85%) had satisfactory pain relief and function for activities of daily living. Return to near normal function was possible for 10 patients who had functional muscle-tendon units.

In 1990, Cofield and Edgerton[17] presented 79 failed arthroplasties that required reoperation. Eight shoulders underwent reoperation for failed constrained shoulder arthroplasty. The remainder required reoperation of failed unconstrained arthroplasties. Numerous factors were identified that led to revision surgery. Unfortunately, the authors did not report the results of most of the patients in this series, presumably due to the heterogeneity of diagnoses and revision procedures performed.

Caldwell and associates[56] reviewed 13 revision arthroplasties with an average follow-up of 36 months. Seven humeral hemiarthroplasties were revised to total shoulder arthroplasty because of glenoid arthrosis, three total shoulder arthroplasties were revised to hemiarthroplasty because of glenoid component loosening, and three arthroplasties (two total and one hemiarthroplasty) were revised because of instability. Results were considered satisfactory in only eight shoulders (62%), and five shoulders needed seven reoperations.

In 1994 and 1996, Wirth and Rockwood[16,38] presented results of 38 consecutive revision arthroplasties. Treatment included 19 total shoulder arthroplasties, 11 hemiarthroplasties, and eight resection arthroplasties. Instability was at least one of the indications for revision in 43% of cases. Twenty-five shoulders, including nine resection arthroplasties, were followed up for a minimum of 2 years. Eight of the nine patients with resection arthroplasties had significant pain relief and could perform limited activities. Of the remaining 16 shoulders, five were graded excellent, seven satisfactory, and four received unsatisfactory grades.

Eighteen patients who underwent revision of a painful hemiarthroplasty to a total shoulder arthroplasty for treatment of glenoid arthrosis were reviewed by Sperling and Cofield[31] in 1998. Diagnoses included trauma (10 shoulders), osteoarthritis (four), rheumatoid arthritis (two), and osteonecrosis secondary to steroids (two). The interval between hemiarthroplasty and the total shoulder arthroplasty averaged 4.4 years. Overall, pain decreased considerably and a significant improvement in motion was seen. However, seven of the 18 shoulders (39%) received an unsatisfactory rating due to limited range of motion or the need for reoperation.

In 1999, Hawkins and associates[22] presented a series of nine patients with symptomatic loose glenoid components who underwent revision arthroplasty. Four of the nine patients had a painful clunk with forward elevation preoperatively. Seven patients underwent reimplantation of another cemented glenoid component, while two underwent removal of the glenoid component. Satisfactory results were seen in seven of the nine patients (78%). Two patients who had reimplantation of a new glenoid component were considered failures due to recurrent loosening.

THE AUTHORS' EXPERIENCE

In 1997, the Shoulder Service at the New York Presbyterian Medical Center presented a series of 50 revision shoulder arthroplasties performed in 50 patients.[57] All patients had a minimum follow-up of 2 years, with a mean of 5 years. Patients averaged 2.5 previous surgeries (range, 1 to 13). The index procedure was total shoulder arthroplasty in 16 (32%) and humeral hemiarthroplasty in 34 (68%). Fifteen of the 50 humeral components were modular in design. The initial diagnosis was severe proximal humerus fracture in 27 patients (54%), osteoarthritis in 10 (20%), osteonecrosis in nine (18%), postcapsulorrhaphy arthropathy in three (6%), and postinfectious arthritis in one (2%).

Causes of prosthetic failures were often multifactorial and included, in order of decreasing frequency, aseptic component loosening, component malposition, instability, rotator cuff pathology, tuberosity malunion or nonunion, soft-tissue contracture, infection, and pain due to glenoid arthrosis. Component loosening was the most common cause of failure of the primary arthroplasty in this series. The glenoid component was loose in 11 patients, and the humeral component was loose in eight. The time interval between initial arthroplasty and revision averaged 36 months (range, 1 to 208 months). In nine patients (18%), a painful humeral hemiarthroplasty was converted to a total shoulder arthroplasty for painful glenoid arthrosis. In five of these, implantation of the glenoid component was facilitated by removal of a modular humeral head. In eight patients (16%), a total shoulder arthroplasty was converted to hemiarthroplasty for failure of a glenoid component. The remaining cases involved exchange of a humeral or glenoid component, or both. The revision procedures performed were tailored according to the specific pathology encountered and often involved a complex reconstruction. Procedures performed in addition to component revision included rotator cuff repair, soft-tissue release, tuberosity reconstruction, coracoacromial arch reconstruction, and deltoidplasty.

Overall, there were 10 excellent (20%), 21 satisfactory (42%), and 19 unsatisfactory results (38%) using Neer's criteria.[48] Eighty-two percent of patients had a significant improvement in their pain. Active postoperative elevation averaged 115°, with an average gain in elevation of 36°. Active external rotation averaged 43°, with an average gain of 21°. Of the eight patients in whom a total shoulder arthroplasty was converted to a hemiarthroplasty, five had a good or excellent result. Of the nine patients in whom a hemiarthroplasty was converted to a total shoulder arthroplasty, five had good or excellent results.

Overall, a high percentage of failures was seen. Patients in the unsatisfactory group had an average of three previous surgeries, compared to 2.5 for the entire study group. Factors associated with failure of the revision procedure included tuberosity malunion or nonunion, instability, perioperative complications, glenoid arthrosis, subscapularis insufficiency, and worker's compensation status. The postoperative complication rate was 20% for the entire series. Complications included three anterior dislocations, two cases of tuberosity displacement, an intraoperative humeral shaft fracture, one wound hematoma, one case of residual anterosuperior instability, one deep prosthetic infection requiring resection arthroplasty, and one case of glenoid component loosening requiring a second revision surgery after 1 year.

The overall success rate was 62%. These results are comparable to those reported by others.[16,19,22,37,39,56] A direct correlation between arthroplasty for proximal humeral fracture and unsatisfactory results was seen, because only 33% satisfactory results were seen in this subset of patients. The poor results seen in the setting of trauma resulted from problems with malunion, nonunion, or resorption of the tuberosities, and contracture of the soft tissues. This result emphasizes the need for careful handling of the soft tissues and secure fixation of the tuberosities at the time of humeral hemiarthroplasty for acute fracture. Half of the patients with instability failed the revision procedure.

In a separate study in 1998, the Shoulder Service at New York Presbyterian Medical Center specifically examined the results of revision of modular humeral components.[58] Advantages of modularity include greater flexibility in matching head size, easier access to the glenoid during revision surgery without the need for removal of the humeral stem, and decreased hospital inventory. Unfortunately, many of the modular designs include a textured surface on the proximal aspect of the humeral stem to improve press-fit or cement fixation or to allow tissue-ingrowth fixation. This aspect of humeral stem design can make removal of the component an extremely difficult and technically challenging operation.

Eleven patients with humeral hemiarthroplasties and six with total shoulder arthroplasties with modular humeral components underwent revision arthroplasty between 1990 and 1996. Follow-up averaged 34 months (range, 12 to 81 months). Thirteen (76%) of the humeral prostheses had been cemented. The humeral component was revised in 10 patients and the modular head was exchanged in the remaining seven. The indications for revision included pain in all cases, instability in six cases, tuberosity nonunion in four cases, glenoid arthrosis in four cases, glenoid component loosening in two cases, and humeral component loosening, severe arthrofibrosis, and infection in one case each. The preoperative range of motion was limited, averaging 72° forward elevation, 11° external rotation, and internal rotation to the L5 vertebral level.

Removal of the humeral component was attempted in all cases. A variety of surgical techniques were used to remove the humeral components including removal of soft-tissue from the proximal bone-prosthesis interface, hammering with a bone tamp and mallet, use of osteotomes down the shaft at the bone-prosthesis or bone-cement interface, a weighted slaphammer attached to the neck of the prosthesis, and humeral shaft osteotomy. After removal of the modular head, use of an extraction device attached to the neck Morse taper can lead to damage of the taper. This can weaken the bond between the taper and a new modular head if stem removal is abandoned. For this reason, the surgeon should be certain that humeral component removal is necessary before using an extraction device attached to the Morse taper.

Overall, two excellent, seven satisfactory, and eight unsatisfactory results were seen using Neer's criteria. Five of the patients with unsatisfactory results had good pain relief but received poor ratings due to limited function. The average gains in forward elevation and external rotation were only 11° and 24°, respectively.

In this series, only four humeral components could be removed without great difficulty. In seven patients, removal of the humeral component was abandoned because of fear that extensive proximal humeral destruction would result with further attempts at implant removal. In these patients, the situation was salvaged by changing the modular head size and balancing the soft-tissues.

Although modularity has definite advantages, revision is difficult because of the proximal textured surface and has the potential for substantial bone loss or fracture. In some instances, it may be necessary to leave a malpositioned prosthesis in place to avoid humeral destruction.

POSTOPERATIVE MANAGEMENT

The postoperative management after revision shoulder arthroplasty is tailored to the patient. Patients who undergo an uncomplicated arthroplasty may be managed in a similar manner to patients who have had a primary shoulder arthroplasty. Typically, this means early passive range-of-motion therapy, beginning on the first day after surgery. Patients requiring revision arthroplasty because of subluxation or dislocation require additional precautions that avoid the position of instability. The position of flexion, adduction, and internal rotation is avoided for 6 weeks in the setting of posterior dislocation, while the position of abduction and external rotation is avoided after anterior dislocations. Patients with a periprosthetic fracture or those who have had a bone grafting procedure may need to be protected for a short period to allow for bone healing.

Active range-of-motion therapy, with the exception of resistive internal rotation, is started about 2 to 3 weeks after surgery. However, active motion is delayed 6 weeks for patients who also had osteotomy and reattachment of a tuberosity.

The risk of joint stiffness is extremely high in this patient population. It is not uncommon for gains in motion and function to occur a year after surgery. Thus, patients should be forewarned preoperatively of the lengthy rehabilitation course.

SUMMARY

Management of failed shoulder arthroplasty is difficult, and the results generally are inferior to results of primary shoulder arthroplasty. Revision shoulder arthroplasty is technically challenging because of the combination of prosthetic failure, bone loss, deltoid or rotator cuff dysfunction, and soft-tissue scarring. Patients often achieve satisfactory pain relief. Unfortunately, significant improvement in range of motion, strength, and function is less predictable. These results underscore the importance of performing a good initial arthroplasty, regardless of the indication. Patients should be educated about the likelihood of achieving a satisfactory result before considering revision shoulder arthroplasty.

REFERENCES

1. Neer CS II: Articular replacement for the humeral head. *J Bone Joint Surg* 1955;37A:215–228.
2. Amstutz HC, Thomas BJ, Kabo JM, Jinnah RH, Dorey FJ: The Dana total shoulder arthroplasty. *J Bone Joint Surg* 1988;70A:1174–1182.

3. Arntz CT, Jackins S, Matsen FA III: Prosthetic replacement of the shoulder for the treatment of defects in the rotator cuff and the surface of the glenohumeral joint. *J Bone Joint Surg* 1993;75A: 485–491.

4. Arntz CT, Matsen FA III, Jackins S: Surgical management of complex irreparable rotator cuff deficiency. *J Arthroplasty* 1991;6:363–370.

5. Barrett WP, Franklin JL, Jackins SE, Wyss CR, Matsen FA III: Total shoulder arthroplasty. *J Bone Joint Surg* 1987;69A:865–872.

6. Brenner BC, Ferlic DC, Clayton ML, Dennis DA: Survivorship of unconstrained total shoulder arthroplasty. *J Bone Joint Surg* 1989;71A: 1289–1296.

7. Cofield RH: Total shoulder arthroplasty with the Neer prosthesis. *J Bone Joint Surg* 1984;66A: 899–906.

8. Fenlin JM Jr, Ramsey ML, Allardyce TJ, Frieman BG: Modular total shoulder replacement: Design rationale, indications, and results. *Clin Orthop* 1994;307:37–46.

9. Gartsman GM, Russell JA, Gaenslen E: Modular shoulder arthroplasty. *J Shoulder Elbow Surg* 1997;6:333–339.

10. Hawkins RJ, Bell RH, Jallay B: Total shoulder arthroplasty. *Clin Orthop* 1989;242:188–194.

11. Kelly IG, Foster RS, Fisher WD: Neer total shoulder replacement in rheumatoid arthritis. *J Bone Joint Surg* 1987;69B:723–726.

12. Levine WN, Djurasovic M, Glasson JM, Pollock RG, Flatow EL, Bigliani LU: Hemiarthroplasty for glenohumeral osteoarthritis: Results correlated to degree of glenoid wear. *J Shoulder Elbow Surg* 1997;6:449–454.

13. Roper BA, Paterson JM, Day WH: The Roper-Day total shoulder replacement. *J Bone Joint Surg* 1990;72B:694–697.

14. Sperling JW, Cofield RH, Rowland CM: Neer hemiarthroplasty and Neer total shoulder arthroplasty in patients fifty years old or less: Long-term results. *J Bone Joint Surg* 1998;80A:464–473.

15. Torchia ME, Cofield RH, Settergren CR: Total shoulder arthroplasty with the Neer prosthesis: Long-term results. *J Shoulder Elbow Surg* 1997;6: 495–505.

16. Wirth MA, Rockwood CA Jr: Complications of total shoulder-replacement arthroplasty. *J Bone Joint Surg* 1996;78A:603–616.

17. Cofield RH, Edgerton BC: Total shoulder arthroplasty: Complications and revision surgery, in Green WB (ed): *Instructional Course Lectures XXXIX*. Park Ridge, IL, American Academy of Orthopaedic Surgeons, 1990, pp 449–462.

18. Matsen FA III, Rockwood CA Jr, Wirth MA, Lippitt SB: Glenohumeral arthritis and its management, in Rockwood CA Jr, Matsen FA III Wirth MA, Harryman DT II (eds): *The Shoulder*, ed 2. Philadelphia, PA, WB Saunders, 1998, vol 2, pp 840–964.

19. Neer CS II, Kirby RM: Revision of humeral head and total shoulder arthroplasties. *Clin Orthop* 1982;170:189–195.

20. Matsen FA III: Early effectiveness of shoulder arthroplasty for patients who have primary glenohumeral degenerative joint disease. *J Bone Joint Surg* 1996;78A:260–264.

21. Petersen SA, Hawkins RJ: Revision of failed total shoulder arthroplasty. *Orthop Clin North Am* 1998;29:519–533.

22. Hawkins RJ, Greis PE, Bonutti PM: Treatment of symptomatic glenoid loosening following unconstrained shoulder arthroplasty. *Orthopedics* 1999;22:229–234.

23. Kelleher IM, Cofield RH, Becker DA, Beabout JW: Fluoroscopically positioned radiographs of total shoulder arthroplasty. *J Shoulder Elbow Surg* 1992;1:306–311.

24. Rafii M, Minkoff J: Advanced arthrography of the shoulder with CT and MR imaging. *Radiol Clin North Am* 1998;36:609–633.

25. Codd TP, Arroyo JS, Flatow EL: Glenoid revision surgery in total shoulder arthroplasty. *Semin Arthroplasty* 1997;8:328–340.

26. Neer CS II (ed): *Shoulder Reconstruction*. Philadelphia, PA, WB Saunders, 1990, pp 143–271.

27. Bonutti PM, Hawkins RJ, Saddemi S: Arthroscopic assessment of glenoid component loosening after total shoulder arthroplasty. *Arthroscopy* 1993;9:272–276.

28. Cofield RH, Chang W, Sperling JW: Complications of shoulder arthroplasty, in Iannotti JP, Williams GR Jr (eds): *Disorders of the Shoulder: Diagnosis and Management.* Philadelphia, PA, Lippincott Williams & Wilkins, 1999, pp 571–593.

29. Shaffer BS, Giordano CP, Zuckerman JD: Revision of a loose glenoid component facilitated by a modular humeral component: A technical note. *J Arthroplasty* 1990;5(suppl):S79–S81.

30. O'Driscoll SW, Petrie R, Torchia M: Arthroscopic glenoid removal for failed total shoulder arthroplasty. *J Shoulder Elbow Surg* 1999;8:665.

31. Sperling JW, Cofield RH: Revision total shoulder arthroplasty for the treatment of glenoid arthrosis. *J Bone Joint Surg* 1998;80A:860–867.

32. Klimkiewicz JJ, Iannotti JP, Rubash HE, Shanbhag AS: Aseptic loosening of the humeral component in total shoulder arthroplasty. *J Shoulder Elbow Surg* 1998;7:422–426.

33. Wirth MA, Agrawal CM, Mabrey JD, et al: Isolation and characterization of polyethylene wear debris associated with osteolysis following total shoulder arthroplasty. *J Bone Joint Surg* 1999;81A:29–37.

34. Codd TP, Yamaguchi K, Pollock RG, Flatow EL, Bigliani LU: Abstract: Infected shoulder arthroplasties: Treatment with staged reimplantation vs. resection arthroplasty. *J Shoulder Elbow Surg* 1996;5:S5.

35. Post M, Pollock RG: Operative treatment of degenerative and arthritic diseases of the glenohumeral joint, in Post M, Bigliani LU, Flatow EL, Pollock RG (eds): *The Shoulder: Operative Technique.* Baltimore, MD, Williams & Wilkins, 1998, pp 73–131.

36. Ramsey ML, Fenlin JM Jr: Use of an antibiotic impregnated bone cement block in the revision of an infected shoulder arthroplasty. *J Shoulder Elbow Surg* 1996;5:479–482.

37. Duncan CP, Masri BA: The role of antibiotic-loaded cement in the treatment of an infection after a hip replacement. *J Bone Joint Surg* 1994;76A:1742–1751.

38. Wirth MA, Rockwood CA Jr: Complications of shoulder arthroplasty. *Clin Orthop* 1994;307:47–69.

39. Moeckel BH, Altchek DW, Warren RF, Wickiewicz TL, Dines DM: Instability of the shoulder after arthroplasty. *J Bone Joint Surg* 1993;75A:492–497.

40. Flatow EL, Weinstein DM, Duralde XA, Compito CA, Pollock RG, Bigliani LU: Abstract: Coracoacromial ligament preservation in rotator cuff surgery. *J Shoulder Elbow Surg* 1994;3:S73.

41. Flatow EL, Connor PM, Levine WN, Arroyo JS, Pollock RG, Bigliani LU: Coracoacromial arch reconstruction for anterosuperior subluxation after failed rotator cuff surgery: A preliminary report. *J Shoulder Elbow Surg* 1997;6:228.

42. Neer CS II, Morrison DS: Glenoid bone-grafting in total shoulder arthroplasty. *J Bone Joint Surg* 1988;70A:1154–1162.

43. Bonutti PM, Hawkins RJ: Fracture of the humeral shaft associated with total replacement arthroplasty of the shoulder: A case report. *J Bone Joint Surg* 1992;74A:617–618.

44. Campbell JT, Moore RS, Iannotti JP, Norris TR, Williams GR: Periprosthetic humeral fractures: Mechanisms of fracture and treatment options. *J Shoulder Elbow Surg* 1998;7:406–413.

45. Groh GI, Heckman MM, Curtis RJ, Rockwood CA Jr: Treatment of fractures adjacent to humeral prosthesis. *Orthop Trans* 1994;18:1072.

46. Boyd AD Jr, Thornhill TS, Barnes CL: Fractures adjacent to humeral prostheses. *J Bone Joint Surg* 1992;74A:1498–1504.

47. Wright TW, Cofield RH: Humeral fractures after shoulder arthroplasty. *J Bone Joint Surg* 1995;77A:1340–1346.

48. Neer CS II, Watson KC, Stanton FJ: Recent experience in total shoulder replacement. *J Bone Joint Surg* 1982;64A:319–337.

49. Flatow EL, Bigliani LU: Tips of the trade: Locating and protecting the axillary nerve in shoulder surgery. The tug test. *Orthop Rev* 1992;21:503–505.

50. Rowe CR: Arthrodesis of the shoulder used in treating painful conditions. *Clin Orthop* 1983;173:92–96.

51. Hawkins RJ, Neer CS III: A functional analysis of shoulder fusions. *Clin Orthop* 1987;223:65–76.

52. Cofield RH, Briggs BT: Glenohumeral arthrodesis: Operative and long-term functional results. *J Bone Joint Surg* 1979;61A:668–677.

53. Richards RR, Beaton D, Hudson AR: Shoulder arthrodesis with plate fixation: Functional outcome analysis. *J Shoulder Elbow Surg* 1993;2:225–239.

54. Neer CS, Brown TH Jr, McLaughlin HL: Fracture of the neck of the humerus with dislocation of the head fragment. *Am J Surg* 1953;85:252–258.

55. Cofield RH: Shoulder arthrodesis and resection arthroplasty, in Stauffer ES (ed): American Academy of Orthopaedic Surgeons *Instructional Course Lectures XXXIV*. St. Louis, MO, CV Mosby, 1985, pp 268–277.

56. Caldwell GL, Dines D, Warren R, Altchek D, Wickiewicz T: Revision shoulder arthroplasty. *Orthop Trans* 1993;17:140–141.

57. Connor PM, Levine WN, Arroyo JS, et al: The surgical management of failed shoulder arthroplasty. *Orthop Trans* 1997;21:6.

58. Arroyo JS, Marra G, Pollock RG, Flatow EL, Bigliani LU: Revision of modular humeral components. *J Shoulder Elbow Surg* 1999;8:188–189.

FUTURE DIRECTIONS

GEOFFREY JOHNSTON, MD AND LOUIS U. BIGLIANI, MD

INTRODUCTION

Over the last decades shoulder arthroplasty has been performed more commonly as the indications for arthroplasty have increased. Through the years the understanding of shoulder anatomy, biomechanics, and function has improved, leading to refinement and evolution of surgical technique. Recent interest in basic science research involving the shoulder joint has stimulated advances in prosthesis technology that benefit shoulder arthroplasty. Orthopaedic surgeons now are able to routinely perform a shoulder replacement for the more straightforward diagnosis and to begin to tackle the more complex reconstructive challenges, which have posed problems for them in the past.

Many different design concepts and prostheses have been introduced in the last 10 years, providing a variety of alternatives from which to choose. This abundance of new information and knowledge, however, can result in confusion as to which is the best choice in a specific instance. Therefore, more than ever, it is imperative to record and communicate experience involving the various aspects of shoulder arthroplasty. Shoulder arthroplasty has enjoyed a relatively high success rate with reference to short-term results. Unfortunately, complications and failures do occur and will continue to increase in the long term. Therefore, in the future orthopaedic surgeons will face the challenge of prosthesis revision, and new technology is needed to overcome these problems.

Shoulder arthroplasty has become a highly technical and precise scientific discipline. Future development and innovation are crucial for progress. This development must be broad-based, encompassing basic science research, such as in the field of material properties of components, and well-organized prospective clinical outcome studies to accurately evaluate results. Shoulder arthroplasty is rapidly progressing in its development. There will be sufficient opportunity to change technique and improve results, providing benefit for patients.

Currently orthopaedic surgeons are in the midst of an evolving third generation of shoulder arthroplasty. Prosthetic adaptability is central to this new concept in shoulder arthroplasty, allowing for correct placement of the prosthetic head, thereby restoring the normal glenohumeral anatomy and kinematics. In this sense, the component incorporates both modularity and an offset head and neck angle. Transition to this generation has been somewhat more cautious because these developments signify substantial change in the design of the prosthesis. It still is believed that the goal of shoulder replacement arthroplasty is to replicate as closely as possible the normal anatomy of the proximal humerus.[3–8] Therefore, because of the offset relationship between the center of rotation of the shaft and the center of rotation of the humeral head, there must be variation of the humeral prosthesis in this regard. Without the ability to vary the orientation, the restoration of normal humeral anatomy during arthroplasty may be constrained by the relatively fixed geometry of existing prosthetic systems. This fixed geometry may lead to failure because there may not be duplication of the proximal humerus anatomy, and this lack may produce abnormal kinematics.

There also is an effort to improve the design and to address the anatomic considerations of the glenoid component. A significant amount of research is being done in reference to pegs versus keels for fixation.[9–11] Additionally, there is interest in improving the articular surface design of the glenoid component. A certain amount of translation in the glenohumeral joint occurs between the humeral head and the glenoid. Normally, the curvature of the glenoid bone is greater than the curvature of the humeral head.[5,12,13] However, normal articulation of the glenohumeral joint actually is highly conformed, because both the thickening of the articular cartilage at the periphery of the glenoid and the presence of the fibrocartilaginous labrum deepen the glenoid, more closely matching its composite curvature to that of the humeral head.[14] Also, the articular cartilage of the humeral head is thicker at its center than at its periphery. This conformity exists for most of the shoulder range of motion in which there is no significant translation, the humeral head remaining centered in the glenoid.[15–18] It is only at the extremes of motion that the humeral head translates more peripherally.[15,19–21] Future designs of the glenoid component should incorporate these anatomic and kinematic considerations to minimize rim- or edge-loading of the prosthesis. Off-center loading on the rim of the glenoid prosthesis may well be the origin of lucent lines and may account for the progression to wider lines and eventual gross loosening of the glenoid component.[4,22–24] There is hope that with the new designs of the humeral head and the glenoid such indices of failure will be decreased substantially.

THE FUTURE

The future of shoulder arthroplasty will be determined by the progress in basic science and clinical research. Notwithstanding the many considerations for prosthetic design, future development of shoulder arthroplasty must also address instrumentation, technique, rehabilitation, and outcomes analysis.

For one reason or another, instrumentation systems for shoulder arthroplasty have not evolved as rapidly as they have for hip and knee arthroplasty. The technical goals of prosthesis placement can be achieved only if the prostheses can be implanted precisely. Precise instrumentation that allows accurate resection of oftentimes deformed bony anatomy, coupled with instruments that facilitate better exposure of the glenoid and humeral head, are required to complement preoperative planning, in order to achieve a reproducible and ultimately successful outcome.

Rehabilitation after shoulder arthroplasty has always been emphasized. However, improvement of the postoperative exercise regimen must continue if the patient is to achieve greater range of motion with minimal pain in the early postoperative period. Furthermore, to achieve maximal function, innovations in the strengthening program must be developed that will predictably fulfil preoperative expectations of gain.

Finally, it is important for orthopaedic surgeons to evaluate that which they have done to help direct them into the future. Recently outcomes' analysis research has gained timely prominence. Without this type of scrutiny surgeons will never know the impact of their work, not only on pain, range of motion, and strength, but also on function and, most importantly, on the quality of their patients' lives. Information from these analyses will allow the surgeons to focus their energies on the identified deficiencies or needs.

The practice of shoulder arthroplasty has matured tremendously over the last century. Orthopaedic surgeons now can effectively treat a wide spectrum of diseases that have caused disabling arthritis of the glenohumeral joint. Individualized preoperative planning, precise implantation of third-generation shoulder prostheses with soft-tissue balancing, and rehabilitation structured to maximize range of motion and strength can optimize the patients' response to surgery. Finally, with both willingness and commitment to participate in outcomes' analysis, orthopaedic surgeons will be able to identify imperfections in approach or implant design, and, through ongoing research, correct these.

Two of Sir Winston Churchill's quotes seem appropriate in describing the evolution of shoulder arthroplasty on the threshold of the new millenium:

"Now this is not the end. It is not even the beginning of the end. But it is, perhaps, the end of the beginning."

"Give us the tools, and we will finish the job."

REFERENCES

1. Neer CS II, Watson KC, Stanton FJ: Recent experience in total shoulder replacement. *J Bone Joint Surg* 1982;64A:319–337.

2. Iannotti JP, Gabriel JP, Schneck SL, Evans BG, Misra S: The normal glenohumeral relationships: An anatomical study of one hundred and forty shoulders. *J Bone Joint Surg* 1992;74A:491–500.

3. Neer CS II: Glenohumeral arthroplasty, in Neer CS (ed): *Shoulder Reconstruction*. Philadelphia, PA, WB Saunders, 1990, pp 143–271.

4. Figgie HE III, Inglis AE, Goldberg VM, Ranawat CS, Figgie MP, Wile JM: An analysis of factors affecting the long-term results of total shoulder arthroplasty in inflammatory arthritis. *J Arthroplasty* 1988;3:123–130.

5. Rietveld AB, Daanen HA, Rozing PM, Obermann WR: The lever arm in glenohumeral abduction after hemiarthroplasty. *J Bone Joint Surg* 1988;70B:561–565.

6. Boileau P, Walch G, Liotard JP: Cineradiographic study of active elevation of the prosthetic shoulder. *J Orthop Surg* 1992;6:351–359.

7. Boileau P, Walch G: The three-dimensional geometry of the proximal humerus: Implications for surgical technique and prosthetic design. *J Bone Joint Surg* 1997;79B:857–865.

8. Iannotti JP, Williams GR: Total shoulder arthroplasty: Factors influencing prosthetic design. *Orthop Clin North Am* 1998;29:377–391.

9. McCullagh PJ: Biomechanics and design of shoulder arthroplasty. *Proc Inst Mech Eng [H]* 1995;209:207–213.

10. Orr TE, Wong BE, Maw K, Ashmore WP, Mason MD: The effect of component fixation design on the performance of glenoid prostheses. *Trans Orthop Res Soc* 1997;22:881.

11. Lacroix D, Murphy LA, Prendergast PJ: Three-dimensional finite element analysis of glenoid replacement prosthese: A comparison of keeled and pegged anchorage systems. *J Biomech Engr*, in press.

12. Soslowsky LJ, Ateshian GA, Mow VC: Stereophotogrammetric determination of joint anatomy and contact areas, in Mow VC, Ratcliffe A, Woo SLY (eds): *Biomechanics of Diarthrodial Joints*. New York, NY, Springer-Verlag, 1990, vol 2, pp 243–268.

13. Soslowsky LJ, Ateshian GA, Bigliani LU, Flatow EL, Mow VC: Sphericity of glenohumeral joint articulating surfaces. *Trans Orthop Res Soc* 1989;14:228.

14. Howell SM, Galinat BJ: The glenoid-labral socket: A constrained articular surface. *Clin Orthop* 1989;243:122–125.

15. Karduna AR, Williams GR, Williams JL, Iannotti JP: Kinematics of the glenohumeral joint: Influences of muscle forces, ligamentous contraints, and articular geometry. *J Orthop Res* 1996;14:986–993.

16. Kelkar R, et al: Glenohumeral kinematics. *JSES* 1993;2(suppl):28.

17. Kelkar R, et al: The effects of articular congruence and humeral head rotation on glenohumeral kinematics. *Adv Bioeng* 1994;28:19–20

18. Poppen NK, Walker PS: Normal and abnormal motion of the shoulder. *J Bone Joint Surg* 1976;58A:195–201.

19. Harryman DT II, Sidles JA, Matsen FA III: Range of motion and obligate translation in the shoulder: The role of the coracohumeral ligament. *Trans Orthop Res Soc* 1990;15:273.

20. Harryman DT II, Sidles JA, Clark JM, McQuade KJ, Gibb TD, Matsen FA III: Translation of the humeral head on the glenoid with passive glenohumeral motion. *J Bone Joint Surg* 1990;72A:1334–1343.

21. Howell SM, Galinat BJ, Renzi AJ, Marone PJ: Normal and adnormal mechanics of the glenohumeral joint in the horizontal plane. *J Bone Joint Surg* 1988;70A:227–232.

22. Friedman RJ: Glenohumeral translation after total shoulder arthroplasty. *J Shoulder Elbow Surg* 1992;1:312–316.

23. Karduna AR, Williams GR, Iannotti JP, Williams JL: Total shoulder arthroplasty biomechanics: A study of the forces and strains at the glenoid component. *J Biomech Eng* 1998;120:92–99.

24. Friedman RJ, An YH, Draughn RA: Glenohumeral congruency in total shoulder arthroplasty. *Orthop Trans* 1997–98;21:17.

INDEX

A
Achilles tendon allografts, 42, 53
acromioclavicular joints, 17
acromion, erosion, 21
acromioplasty, 53
activities of daily living, 47
adhesions, 28, 54
alcoholism, 20
Amstutz, Harlan C., 5
anesthesia, 27-28
ankylosis, 2
anterior instability, 42, 53
anteroposterior radiographs
   indications for revision, 48
   osteoarthritis, 27
   postoperative, 35
   preoperative, 27
   rotator cuff-tear arthropathy, 22
   stage V osteonecrosis, 21
antibiotics
   impregnated beads, 43, 43
   parenteral, 43
   prophylactic, 51
arthritis. see also Osteoarthritis
   capsulorrhaphy, 21
   glenohumeral, 13, 21-23
   postinfectious, 58
   rheumatoid, 19
   septic, 22
   shoulder, 18
   traumatic, 19
arthrodeses, 22-23
arthrography, 49
arthroplasty, 2, 4, 57
arthroscopy, 49
arthroses, 51
articular cartilage, 17, 18, 66
aseptic loosening, 44-45, 51
axillary nerves
   identification, 29-30
   injury, 40-41
   revision surgery, 54-55
   "tug test," 29, 29, 55
axillary radiographs, 27
   glenohumeral wear, 27
   glenoid component loosening, 50
   glenoid erosion, 53
   humeral head, 35
   indications for revision, 48

B
Baer, William, 2
ball and socket appliances, 7, 10
Bankart retractors, 31, 32
Barton, John Rhea, 2
Bateman appliances, 6
beach chair position, 28, 54
Bickel appliances, 7, 9, 10
Bipolar appliances, 6, 13
bone
   glenoid stock, 49
   humeral, 51
   quality, 55
   resorption, 43
   severe loss, 22
bone grafting, 43, 52, 54
bursa, 28

C
C-reactive proteins, 49
capsular plication, 53
capsulectomy, 45
capsules, 30, 34
captured ball and socket appliances, 10
cement
   antibiotic impregnated, 51
   and glenoid wear, 33
   humeral implantation, 34
   nerve injury, 41
   placement, 32, 34
   postoperative radiograph, 35
   protrusion, 45
   radiolucencies, 43, 44-45, 49
   removal, 43, 55
cephalic veins, 54
cerclage wires, 40, 54, 55
cerviocromial ligaments, 43-44
Charcot joints, 13
Charnley, John, 3-4
chondroitin sulfate, 22
Clarke, Ian, 5
Clayton spacer, 6, 8
cloud treatment, 44
compliance, patient, 49
complications
   need for revision, 48
   postoperative, 41-46
   revision shoulder arthroplasty, 59
   total shoulder arthroplasty, 39-46
components. see also Specific components
   loosening, 48, 58
   malpositioning, 41, 42
computed tomography scans, 49
constrained prostheses, 7, 9-13
contact activity, 35
contractures
   coracohumeral ligaments, 54
   long-term, 45
   release, 45, 55
   traumatic arthritis, 19
coracohumeral ligaments, 54
coracoid strap muscles, 55
coracromial arch, 53
coracromial ligament resection, 53
corticosteroids, 20
"crescent" signs, 20
Cruess classification, 20-21
cup arthroplasties, 2, 3, 6
cysts, 18

D
DANA (designed after natural anatomy), 5, 6, 8
deAnquin, C.E., 3
delamination, 50
Delta III appliances, 7, 9, 11, 12
deltoid muscles, 53
   atony, 53
   dysfunction, 19, 41, 48
   scarring, 55
deltoid myofascial facial sleeve, 34
deltopectoral approach, 28-30, 54
digital subtraction techniques, 49
dislocations, 21, 41, 53
drills, 55

dysbarism, 20

E
edge loading, 53
education, patient, 39, 49
elbow, 17
electrocautery, needlepoint, 55
electromyography (EMG), 41
Englebrecht, E., 4
English-MacNab appliances, 6
epinephrine, 33
erosion
　acromion, 21
　glenoid, 18, 19, 53
　humeral head, 19
exercises, postoperative, 35
experience, prevention of complications, 39

F
fascial flaps, 2
Fenlin, J.M. Jr., 13
Fenlin appliances, 7, 9, 11, 13
Floating Socket appliances, 7, 9, 11
fluoroscopic guidance, 49
follow-up visits, 35
fracture-dislocations, comminuted, 3
fracture orthosis, 54
fracture plate fixation, 40
fractures
　fixation, 40
　intraoperative, 39-40, 54
　periprosthetic, 48, 54
　prosthesis tip, 44
　proximal humerus, 52, 54, 56
fusion, glenohumeral, 57

G
Gaucher's disease, 20
glass, 2
glenohumeral joints
　abduction, 18
　AP radiograph, 27
　arthritis, 13, 21-23
　arthrodesis, 22-23
　fusion, 57
　motion, 17
　posterior instability, 18
　relationships, 17
glenoid
　articular surface, 18
　attachment, 17
　axillary view, 27
　cement penetration, 40

components, 31, 33
erosion, 21, 53
exposure, 30
inspection, 31
intraoperative fractures, 40
penetration of canal, 40
posterior wear, 42, 49
preparation, 32
surface erosion, 18, 19
wear, 4, 33
glenoid arthrosis, 51, 58
glenoid component loosening
　aseptic, 44-45
　axillary radiograph, 50
　bone resorption, 43
　and edge loading, 53
　incidence, 23, 44, 58
　need for revision, 36, 49
　reoperation for, 4
glenoid components
　arthroscopy, 49
　implantation, 31-34
　removal, 50
　wear, 50
glenoid fossa, 20
glenoidplasties, 5
Gluck, Thermistockles, 1
glucosamine, 22
granulation tissue, 19
greater tuberosities, 17, 21, 35
Gristina appliances, 5, 6, 8

H
headrests, 28
hemiarthroplasty, 36, 51, 52
hemostasis, 33
heterotopic ossification, 45
history, total shoulder athroplasties, 1-15
humeral circumflex arteries, 29
humeral components
　anteversion, 53
　history, 3
　implantation, 34
　loosening, 36, 45, 50-51
　superior migration, 42, 44
humeral heads
　articular surface, 17
　aseptic loosening, 50
　dissociation, 45
　erosions, 19
　height, 34-35, 52
　history, 3
　modular, 58
　offset prostheses, 41
　osteonecrosis, 20

osteotomy, 30
position, 17
postoperative radiograph, 35
replacements, 47
size, 30, 34, 42
translation, 30
humeral shaft
　fracture classification, 54
　intraoperative fracture, 39-40
humerus
　canal diameter, 27
　cortical thinning, 19
　extended osteotomy, 51
　fracture-dislocations, 3
　loss of normal height, 42
　preparation, 30-31
　proximal fractures, 42, 45, 54, 56, 58
　reaming, 30
　restoration of length, 54
　superior migration, 53
　wear, 27
hypertrophic synovitis, 50

I
Iannotti, Joseph, 13
immobilization, fractures, 54
immunosuppressive medications, 22
implants. see also Specific components
　aseptic loosening, 44-45
　dissociation, 45-46
　frequency of complications, 39
　indications for revision, 48
　position in serial radiographs, 49
　removal in infection, 43
incidences
　capsulorrhaphy arthritis, 21
　component instability, 41-42
　glenoid loosening, 23, 44, 58
　intraoperative fractures, 39
　intraoperative nerve injury, 40
　osteoarthritis, 18
　osteonecrosis, 20
　postoperative rotator cuff tear, 43
　rheumatoid arthritis, 19
　rotator cuff tears, 19
　superior migration, 42
　traumatic arthritis, 19
incisions, deltopectoral, 28, 54
infections
　component loosening, 43
　indications for revision, 48,

49, 51-52
  postoperative, 43
inferior capsule release, 55
inferior instability, postoperative, 42-43, 53-54
inflammation, 19
instability. *see also* Specific components
  anterior, 53
  chronicity, 53
  of components, 41-42
  glenohumeral, 52-54
  posterior, 53
instrumentation, future of, 66
internal rotation stretching, 35
interposition arthroplasty, 2
intraoperative complications, 39-41
intraoperative fractures, 39-40, 54
Isoelastic appliance, 6

J
Jónsson, E., 2
Jónsson appliances, 6
Jónsson shoulder cup, 3
Judet, R., 3

K
Kessel appliances, 7, 9, 11-12
Köbel appliances, 7, 9-10

L
lifting, postoperative, 35
Liverpool appliances, 7, 9, 11-12
loading, off-centered, 66
long-stem prostheses, 40, 54
loosening. *see* Specific components

M
MacAusland, Andrew, 2
MacNab appliances, 6
magnetic resonance imaging, 20
malpositioning, 41, 42, 53, 56
malunion, 19, 48
manipulation, postoperative stiffness, 45
Mazas appliance, 6, 8
metallosis, 50
methotrexate, 22
Michael Reese appliances, 7, 9, 10
Michaels, J. Porter, 1
Model BME appliances, 7, 9, 10
modular components, 45-46, 58,
60, 65
Monospherical appliances, 5, 6, 8
Morse taper components, 45-46, 59
Murphy, John B., 2
musculocutaneous nerves, 41

N
neck, neutral position, 28
Neer, Charles S. II, 3
Neer fixed-fulcrum arthroplasty, 57
Neer hooded appliances, 6
Neer I appliances, 3, 4
Neer II appliances, 4, 5, 6, 57
Neer Mark III appliances, 7, 9, 11
Neer phases of rehabilitation, 35
Neer prostheses, outcomes, 36
nerve injuries, 19, 40-41
nonconstrained prosthesis, 13
nonsteroidal anti-inflammatory medications, 22, 49
nonunion, 19, 44, 48, 52
nutritional supplementation, 22

O
offset humeral head component, 41
O'Leary-Walker appliances, 6
Ollier, Louis Xavier Edouard Leopold, 2
oscillating saws, 30
ossification, posterior heterotopic, 45
osteoarthritis, 18-19
  AP view, 27
  endoprosthetic replacement, 23
  press-fit stem, 34
  revision shoulder arthroplasty, 58
  shoulder, 18
  subscapularis release, 34
  total shoulder arthroplasty, 36
osteolysis, 49, 50
osteomyelitis, 22
osteonecrosis, 20-21, 23, 58
osteopenia, 19, 22
osteophytes, 18, 21
  AP view, 27
  formation, 18
  in osteoarthritis, 18
  peripheral, 31
  removal, 30

osteoporosis, 19, 34
osteotomies
  extended humeral, 51
  humeral head, 30, 31
  repair, 56
  revision surgery, 55
  traumatic arthritis, 19
outcomes
  revision soldier arthroplasty, 57-60
  and surgical technique, 27-37
outlet view, 27

P
pain
  indications for revision, 48, 49
  infection, 49
  outcomes of revision surgery, 47
  relief, 36
  shoulder sympathectomy, 22
pannus, formation, 19
patient histories, 48
patient selection, 39, 48, 49
Péan, Jules Emile, 1
Péan prostheses, 1
periprosthetic fractures, 48, 54
physical examination, 48
physical therapy, 22, 49
polyethylene, 4, 50
positioning, 27-28, 54
Post, Melvin, 10
postcapsulorraphy, 58
posterior dislocation, 42
posterior instability, 42, 53
postinfectious arthritis, 58
postoperative complications, 41-46
postoperative management, 60
postoperative radiographs, 50
postoperative rehabilitation, 35
preoperative planning, 39, 48-49
press-fit fixation, 33, 34
prosthetic adaptability, 65
pulse lavage, 33

R
radial nerve injury, 41
radiographs
  follow-up visits, 35
  indications for revision, 48-49
  osteoarthritis, 18
  preoperative, 27
  prosthesis position, 45
  rheumatoid arthritis, 19
  serial, 48

radiolucent lines, 43-45, 49
range of motion, 36, 48
range-of-motion exercises, 35
reaming
    glenoid, 40
    glenoid version, 31
    humeral shaft, 30
    spherical, 45
rehabilitation, 35, 42
reoperation, frequency of, 47
resection arthroplasty, 22, 57
resisted exercises, 35
retractors, 31
reversed ball and socket appliances, 7, 11-13
revision shoulder arthroplasty, 47-63
    complications, 59
    inferior instability, 42
    outcomes, 57-60
    posterior instability, 42
    postoperative management, 60
    specific indications, 49-54
    surgical techniques, 54-57
rheumatoid arthritis, 19
"rocking horse" movements, 23, 42, 44
rotator cuff
    arthropathy, 21
    compromise, 52
    impingement, 41
    inspection, 29
    outcomes, 36
    tendon rupture, 52
rotator cuff tears, 56
    arthrography, 49
    arthropathy, 22
    indications for revision, 48
    osteoarthritis, 18-19
    outlet view, 27
    postoperative, 42-44
revision surgery, 47
rheumatoid arthritis, 19

S
scapula, bolster under, 28
scapular body, 17
scapular "Y" radiographs, 27, 48
scapulothoracic joints, 17
scarring, 19, 48
scintigraphy, 20
sedimentation rates, 49
semiconstrained prostheses, 6, 8-9, 13
septic arthritis, 22
Shenk, Thomas, 13
shoulder arthroplasty, 27-37

shoulder girdle, 17
shoulders
    anatomy and physiology, 17-18
    indications for arthroplasty, 17-25
Sialstic cup, 2
sickle cell disease, 20
skin flaps, 54
Smith-Peterson, Marius Nygaard, 2
Smith-Peterson Hip Cups, 3
soft-tissue adhesions, 48
soft-tissue balancing, 34-35, 45, 53
soft-tissue repair, 53
soft-tissue sleeve length, 52
soft tissues
    excessive tension, 21
    frequency of complications, 39
    in rheumatoid arthritis, 19
    scarring, 19
sponges, 33
spot radiographs, 49
St. Georg appliances, 4-6, 8
Stanmore appliances, 7, 9, 10
Stellbrink, G., 4-5
sternoclavicular joints, 17
steroids, 19, 20, 22
stiffness, postoperative, 45
strength measurements, 48
subacromial space, decompression, 52
subchondral bone plate, 45
subchondral glenoid cysts, 19
subchondral sclerosis, 18
subluxation, 41, 53
subscapularis muscle, 34
subscapularis tendon
    anterior instability, 42
    dehiscence, 53
    length, 34, 55
    reattachment, 35
    repair, 30
    superior transposition, 53
superior glenoid rim, 53
superior migration, humeral, 42, 44, 52, 53
superior subluxation, 43
surgical technique, 27-37
Swanson appliances, 6
sympathectomy, shoulder, 22
systemic lupus erythematosus, 20

T
total shoulder arthroplasty
    complications, 39-46

    future directions, 65-68
    history, 1-15
    indications, 17-25
    revisions, 47-63
    surgical technique, 27-37
Total Shoulder Systems, classification, 4
traction, 54
transosseous sutures, 55
traumatic arthritis, 19
Tri-spherical appliances, 7, 9, 12
trial components, 54
"tug tests," 29, 55

U
ultrasonic cement removal devices, 55
unconstrained systems, 4-6, 47
University of California at Los Angeles (UCLA) total shoulder, 5, 6, 8

V
Varian, J.P.W., 2
Varian appliances, 6
Vitallium, 2

W
wear
    axillary radiographs, 27
    cement, 33
    glenoid, 33, 42, 49, 50
    humeral, 27
weight training, 35
white blood cell count, 49

Z
Z-plasty, 45, 55